Clinical Depression - Unleashing the Terminator

I0118160

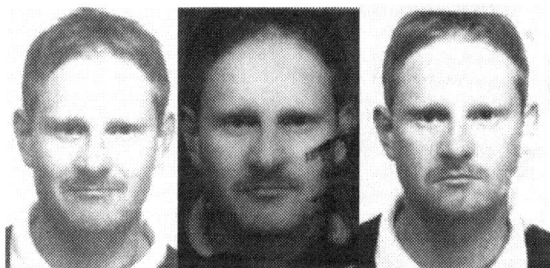

BY David Raymond Jordan

'One Million people commit suicide every year'
The World Health Organization

Published by:
Chipmunkapublishing
PO Box 6872
Brentwood
Essex
CM13 1ZT
United Kingdom

www.chipmunkapublishing.com

Proof-read by Flora Wong

Synopsis

Within the brain of every complex living thing exists a powerful and lethal facility. It is a defence system but it is unlike any other defence for its purpose is not self preservation but self destruction. Because the brain has progressed from simpler origins and has been designed for a life in the natural world the defence can be triggered into action innapropriate circumstances, giving rise to the destructive, terrible and highly misunderstood illness clinical depression.

This is the story of how, through naivity and misfortune, I transgressed from a normal healthy young man stood at life's launch pad into the nightmare of clinical mental illness. It tells of how after 3 years of psychiatric treatment I was left a destroyed, disabled and unemployed person on the scrap heap despite a relentless campaign of resiliance and self help. It also tells of my attempts to get justice for what I believed to be medical negligence, and how self love and fighting spirit would never let me give up my goal to regain my health, future and well being.

As well as describing (and I believe indisputably explaining) clinical depression this book also contains my views on evolution, religion, civilisation, animal rights, anxiety illness, the psychiatric system and world population growth, re-molded and revisited by my terrible experiences, continuing education and progressing maturity.

I truly wish I had the knowledge contained in this book when I was aged 20, for it would have saved me from a disaster. I believe that if my book is widely read it will save lives and save some from going through the excessive suffering that I did, as well as giving people an insight into the realities and true nature of mental illness. This may increase empathy for the mentally ill. The occurance of this illness is a statistical inevitability yet it's nature is shrouded in misunderstanding. This is my main motivation for writing it. I hope it also encourages people to show more respect for the lives of other living things. I believe my book explains the true nature of life and its inner workings, which persons of a religeous persuasion may find offensive, but more hopefully challenging. My book may even advance medical knowledge.

I have a high standard of education and I have a good Honours degree. I have an interest in natural history, biology and medical issues. I am unashamedly a former psychiatric patient who unfortunately had a very long time to look at and understand his problems. I have worked in the Civil Service for 8 years and as a Manager in Local Government for 11 years.

I feel my book would be of general interest to the population. I think the title is eye catching and evokes curiosity. In my book I have attacked the medical profession. I feel justified in this. This could stimulate debate about the nature of mental illness and the quality of treatment and care for the mentally ill. It raises questions about patient's rights and the accountability of Psychiatrists –and their competence. It could prompt discussion on TV, radio and in papers and magazines. I would be happy to discuss my experiences and opinions in the media. There will be many people who have had this illness (probably without really understanding it), or have relatives who have had it or have lost friends or relatives to it. These people may want to raise their voice in public.

I am not an experienced writer and as I make my living in other ways I have had to put this work together in my spare time. It has been written and modified intermittently over a small number of years and may therefore appear a little disjointed. I am happy to have my account ghost re-written by a more experienced writer.

CLINICAL DEPRESSION – UNLEASHING THE TERMINATOR

So far so good.

I was aged 20 and working in the Department of Health and Social Security as a clerical officer. I had recently moved to the long-term benefits section and was learning the ropes. Behind me sat a pretty girl called Suzanne, the same age as me and quite bright. She helped me out with a lot of my problems. I had a high opinion of her. I thought she would marry a Doctor or somebody high up in society one day though she had a long-standing boyfriend who was much older. He was always ringing her and sending her huge bunches of flowers. I had only two regular friends, Cliff and Steve, but we always went out together at weekends. Things were pretty stable at home. We had a dog called Buster aged nine. I had a black Ford Capri which I would spend hours cleaning and polishing.

I didn't particularly like the DHSS but I didn't really know what to do. I had under performed at secondary school and had joined the Civil Service at age 17. But I had continued my education at night school and had gained some good O'level grades and an A' level in politics. I was now studying psychology A' level which I enjoyed. I was very committed to my course. I used to look through psychology books in the university library and occasionally see articles about depression. 'Who are these people?' I would ask

7

myself. 'If I was feeling that way I would just dig deep and pull myself together'.

At work things were changing. It dawned on me that Suzanne liked me. I would have her in hysterics with my antics and wit. I started to like her too. The worst time of the week became Friday night, because I would not be seeing her again for two days. Meanwhile my friend Cliff got fixed up with a girl called Debbie, and Steve got involved with a girl called Janet. My grandparents died which separated me from my cousins to some extent and our dog buster went missing. Suzanne was making hints that I should ask her out, but I was always waiting for the next best opportunity. I was afraid of getting it wrong and losing her as a friend. After all, the other positive aspects of my life were crumbling. Suzanne was the only thing in my life which brought me any happiness. And then there was that older well-established and very keen boyfriend. She dropped the best hint yet and I didn't act. Suzanne went on holiday – with him – and I awaited her return. Mrs Thatcher was reducing the size of the Civil Service and re-organization was starting to make the office a mad house, phones blazing all day, never enough time to do anything.

The turning point.

When Suzanne returned from holiday things were
different. 'Stop bugging me' she said. That was a
turning point. I guess I knew what it meant and I
started to feel bad. I became irritable and exhausted. I
took my fatigue to be down to a lack of fitness and I
started jogging. I was always tense. I went to see a
horror film at the pictures. I always enjoyed such films
but afterwards I felt somewhat disturbed for the first
time. I went boating with Cliff, Debbie and her sister
Vanessa and I remember feeling that no matter what,
things just wouldn't be right. Suzanne was moved
away from her section to work on producing algorithms
for the purposes of multiskilling a reduced workforce. I
would buy sweets every Friday so I had an excuse to go
and give her some. But there was no reconciliation.
She was cold. My window of opportunity that I had
assumed would be around for a lot longer was gone.
I'd blown it.

At the Christmas party we took to the dance floor. She
told me to find a nice girl for myself. I told her I didn't
understand. She repeated her statement and I said I still
didn't understand. Basically she had made her bed
elsewhere and was brushing me off. During my
Christmas break I felt absolutely terrible. I had time
off, but nobody to do anything with. I despairingly told
myself 'you're being left behiend'. I began to feel like
I was all alone on a raft in the middle of the ocean,

hopelessly lost. I had a sense of impending doom. I felt like I was going to die.

Next month I was sat behind Suzanne and I asked her what she was doing that weekend. 'Why' she asked. 'Because I wondered if you.wanted to go out ' I spluttered, belatedly trying to correct my errors. 'Well I can't really can I' she replied. I felt terrible. I lost my humor and began feeling vacant. It should have been obvious to anyone who knew me that I was deeply troubled. My friend Cliff told me that he had suffered anxiety after splitting from a girlfriend and had 'sorted himself out' in the gym. I would go to the gym to do weights but during my workout I would get a searing pain as if an axe had been driven down the middle of my head and my head would pound all night. My limbs would fly out on their own accord when I relaxed and my back would arch up off the bed as if I had been electrocuted. I felt constantly exhausted. I passed my A'level psychology course with a grade A.

I went for long walks and would end up sitting under motorway bridges just wanting to shut the world out. Everything meant nothing. I felt absolutely terrible. My nerves were all over the place. I knelt over my bed just trying..trying to pull myself together..but I couldn't. I began to have a strong urge to place my clenched hands in front of my face. I realized that I must have some form of depression but I was trying to think and fight my way out of it. I didn't understand why I didn't want to live anymore and why I couldn't pull myself together. I would go to church on my own (outside of mass) and tears would roll down my face. What was happening to me? Why couldn't I beat it? Why didn't I want to live anymore? I would constantly review my past. 'Was it because of this'..'was it because of that..?' 'Did I have Schizophrenia?' I felt absolutely terrified, like something inside was screaming out. I prayed to God for help but none was forthcoming. My confidence and energy levels were so incredibly low, just a few percent of normal. It was as if the life and the will to live were being sucked out of me.   Like I was bleeding to death – but it wasn't blood that was seeping from me, but mental life. I went to see my GP but ended up seeing a junior Doctor. 'Why are you depressed'? he asked impatiently as if I was some sort of malingering weakling. He prescribed me some sleeping pills which made no difference. I went to see a psychotherapist privately but to no avail. He took pictures of my iris as he said he could determine the problem from the stresses therein! I had no energy. I would just lie on the bare floor not wanting to get up. 'What's the point' I would despairingly scream inside. 'What's the point (of living) when we are all going to die one day anyway'. The world had become a different place altogether – hopeless, terrifying, meaningless, futile. The sense of continuity I had experienced all my life was gone. This was something else. This was not planet earth any more. There was an awesome force inside me. It was unlike anything else I had ever experienced. A uni-directional force, massive and overwhelming, taking me somewhere from which there could be no possible return. Somehow everything in life is reversible, everything in life can be undone. Everything has two directions. But not this. This was an awesome one way journey from which it was completely and utterly impossible to return. And it was winning. For all my resistance I was being consumed irreversibly into a vaccum. Eventually I went to see my GP. I told him my problems and experiences. After three visits he suggested I see a psychiatrist and I agreed.

'Help' at last.

I met a policewoman on a motorway bridge. We had a
brief chat. She told me I didn't look very well. She
was right. I went on holiday on my own on an 18-30
holiday. I met a girl called Sally. I tried so hard to act
normal. When she left me at the end of the night tears
would fall. I could not stop this terrible thing that was
happening. I hadn't the strength to do what she wanted
of me. More long crisis walks with me always asking
myself the critical question 'do I want to carry on
living?'. I had to wait another 3 horrible weeks until
my appointment came at the psychiatric out patient's
clinic. I was summoned to a room and told to sit on a
wooden stool. (no comfortable couch in sight) 'What
do you think about being here?', asked the stern and
beetroot faced Dr. Callan. 'Well I'd rather not be here
(silly, cocky and immaturely) but.. I've written this out,
please read it'. I gave him four sides of A4 outlining
my life and my symptoms. He studied in silence then
came to a swift conclusion. 'Well it's not the type you
would get much sympathy for… still it's real, it's
exhaustive and…not very pleasant'. '*No it's not very
pleasant*' I screamed back at him. 'How could you let
a girl do this to you, you win some you loose some.
You're obviously very shy and afraid of rejection'. I
told him I couldn't think straight and was this
psychomotor slowing.? 'No, retardation is caused
by..(can't remember). Mechanisms…. The anxiety
comes first, then the depression. There are two things
to do here, firstly to get rid of the depression, which we

can do easily enough. Secondly to find ways of making sure it doesn't happen again, try to find ways of making you mature, because you're not very mature are you?' 'I have to be honest, there's no point in me being here if I'm not honest'. 'You've got to think..where you went wrong'. All in all it was the biggest dressing down I have ever had, unfairly or otherwise. I told him that I didn't sit there getting depressed and giving up. 'I'll go along with that he said'. 'It's all right, it's only a bit of anxiety, it's nothing to be ashamed of'. Dr. Callan wrote out my prescription of Bolvidon 30mg, told me how to take it and referred me to a high level psychologist. She referred to my pessimism as 'the black cloud'. She said when people say they have been depressed they really mean they have felt low for a couple of hours but I will be able to say that I've had the real thing. (*Well Fucking 'A'*. If I had survived being run over by a lorry I would hardly want to brag about that either.) She said she always noticed tension in patients and gave me a relaxation tape and technique, involving alternately tensing and relaxing all the muscles of the body.

I didn't know what was wrong with me but, aged 22, I thought that all Doctors were competent and caring and that I would be in good hands. I had faith in Doctors, society and the NHS. I continued to work with my pills (never being advised otherwise) hoping that my agony would come to an end. And it was agony. Like a terminally ill person I genuinely wanted to die. I had a massive urge to commit suicide. I was completely out on my feet, bewildered, confused and engulfed in feelings and sensations which were the quite simply the ultimate in terrifying and revolting - feelings and sensations both from beyond the grave and straight out of the abattoir. I could say I felt like a zombie but it seemed worse than that because a zombie would presumably have retained some sense of humanity, which I didn't. I was beyond a zombie. I felt like a living carcass – a slab of meat that had escaped from the back door of a butchers shop, or something that had been dead for years, dug up and brought back to life to what was left of it. My experiences were beyond human words but the best I can do is say it was the most ugly, terrifying, devastating and undesirable experience possible. Something I truly wouldn't have wished upon Hitler. It's power was massive, totally overwhelming. This was unadulterated inhumanity – I was living in Hell. I felt I was at the outer limits of endurance just about hanging onto my existence, whilst experiencing the combined psychology's of extinction and physical annihilation. I could only envisage burning to death being worse than this. If someone had given me £20M I would genuinely have given it all back just to get away from this. The ugliest and most terrifying monster imaginable was alive inside of me, and trying with awesome persuasion to take me away forever. There comes a point in suffering where money is just paper, and I was most definitely at it. Some '*bit of anxiety*'. It wasn't hard to understand why severe depression drives patients to suicide, it seemed very much the thing to do since going through something this terrible was more than life could ever be worth. Whilst I was ill a young man with depression stood in front of a train less than a mile from where I lived. The mother of a girl at work poured petrol over herself and set it alight, dying of her injuries later. A woman living not too far away cut her own throat with a circular saw. Apparently the most seriously ill patients may only attempt suicide three months into treatment – when they have regained enough strength to do so. Dr. Callan was right - severe depression is not very pleasant at all. Severe depression is horrific – it's a journey into the very bowels of Hell. But what exactly is it? What could be so appalling, so immense and overpowering that it could make someone stand in front of a speeding train?

Under treatment.

The drugs hit me like a freight train. I began to slur. Every day I felt like a team of horses were pulling me back to bed. But I got up and went to work – poleaxed and out on my feet. I would go behind the aviary at home, clench my fists and scream inside, 'I'm going to win – two more months, just two more months and you will be ok, you can take it for two more months.' And the months rolled on. I had gruesome nightmares every few weeks. Massacres, killer whales, giant snakes, decapitation, plane crashes, vampires. I took these to be the result of the interaction between the illness and the drug. The theme was always the same – carnage, horror, and death. My suffering just seemed to continue largely unabated. I was referred to Dr. Callan again after seven months and my prescription was doubled. 'We double the dose' he said. I told him I was under a lot of pressure at work and he said it would not do me any permanent harm. As the weeks and months rolled on I began to formulate a conclusion about what had happened, what had gone wrong inside my head. Whilst this conclusion required radical thinking it became undeniable, consistent with all of my experiences and consistent with the world I could now understand differently around me. I do remember describing my depression at an early stage as 'inverted survival instincts' to the psychologist. This wasn't a bad first effort. In hindsight it was pretty close to the mark…Within three months of starting treatment I believe I had correctly unmasked the terrible monster within....

A terrifying, utterly devastating and unstoppable one way force.. like _nothing_ else in this world, irreversibly bleeding the life and will to live out of me. Loss of control of my own mind. An existence which now seemed completely undesirable – and utterly futile. Upon being medicated... sensations of horror, sensations from beyond the grave, sensations from the darkest corners of the abattoir - the most ugly and undesirable sensations possible. Gruesome nightmares, morbidity, mental retardation, '_mechanisms_...' A terrible sense of fear and a sense of affinity with any death and carnage I saw around me. (ie dead animals) What was my 'depression'? What was this massive 'heart attack' taking place inside my head...? The following is my own explanation, based on my experiences, intelligent reasoning and observations of the living world. So confidant am I that it is correct that I welcome anyone of _any_ standing to try to defeat it or put forward a more plausible explanation. For me it fits like a glove.

The Terminator – Standard issue defence.

We are all a little bit different (all species show genetic variation) but essentially how we are made is pretty much standard amongst humans and indeed much to an extent other complex living things: heart, liver, kidneys, eyes, blood, central nervous system, skin, lungs etc.. Religion can't give an adequate answer for this but Darwinian evolution can. Charles Darwin explained that this was because evolution consisted of descent with modification giving rise to a likeness between all living things. All mammals have a common ancestor. All vertebrates have a common ancestor. This is shown in the fossil record – the history of life preserved in rocks. Every living thing on the planet today can trace its origin through an unbroken series of events over 3 ½ billion years. New species are simply an adaptation of what has existed before to a new ecological niche. Over the vastness of time new species have developed to fill all the ecological niches – from the stock of existing species (called adaptive radiation). For example, a polar bear is simply a grizzly bear that has adapted to a life in a cold environment. Within a species there is genetic variation, but this is small compared to the similarities. Natural selection acts on genetic variation and gene mutations to ultimately refine a species or develop a new one. These processes cannot clearly be seen in any one lifetime. Evolution does not have a direction or an end game, (Richard Dawkins describes it as a 'blind watchmaker') it is simply an opportunity to survive taken in a crowded and competative world. Nature selects winning genes by the act of surviving long enough to reproduce. The I am coming to is this, I had found out a little too late that something else comes as a standard issue to living things. Something which was driving this illness to it's conclusion. Something all humans have inherited through the evolutionary line by descent with modification. It's something that you strangely won't find in the biology books, but is an essential component of all living things on our planet – and for good reason....

At a primitive, unconscious and essentially involuntary level the brain (mine, yours and every advanced living thing) is equipped with a *standard* defence mechanism. It is an ultimate defence. It is for the purposes of self-termination in hopeless, horrific or disastrous circumstances. Every complex living thing has this facility as surely as it has a hypothalamus, a pituitary gland, pons, pineal gland a cerebellum and all the other standard bits and pieces. It is part and parcel of being a living thing. Impersonal, unconscious, primordial, beyond voluntary intervention and by deliberate design unstoppable and lethal. Once it kicks in there is no natural way of stopping it running it's course. This awesome genie won't go back into it's bottle. It is not another *inner* person. Just impersonal biological machinery that blindly works the way it has been designed to. A componant part of every complex living thing. This is the *mechanism* that Dr. Callan was referring to. From mice to mammoths and men, flesh and blood is universally equipped with the ultimate defence facility – as standard. This is a necessity for a life on our planet and it's existance helps to bring home the true nature of life on earth. All it needs is the right stimulus to spring into action – to do its job, which it blindly does. Little wonder that I felt like I was going to die – because short of psychiatric medicine I was. I could not voluntarily stop it, it was never designed to be stopped. For all my defiance and resiliance it was getting stronger and I was getting weaker. Yet as terrible as it is, it is in fact nature's mercy in the face of the unimaginable, when the end of your days or things even worse are inevitable. In the circumstances for which it was designed it is your greatest ally. My brain was now divided into a conscious confused persona and a primitive impersonal unconscious heading full steam for eternity. But at the time I didn't know what was happening to me, how or why.

Taking a close look around at life on earth it is not hard to realise why it is so appropriate for nature (or God for those who prefer) to endow its creations with such a defence. We may spend most of our lives living in a comfort zone (and in the case of humans at the more privileged end of a food chain) but no living thing is immune from disaster. Every living thing on our planet is a physical and mortal entity. All will fail eventually, but many lives are destined to be cut short, potentially in the most brutal and cruel circumstances. The world can dramatically change, often in an instant. The reality of life on earth is that it can deliver the most terrible, brutal and appalling outcomes to any of its physical inhabitants – and it very frequently does. The physical destruction of complex living things on our planet is a very common occurrence, taking place on a massive scale every day. This we can see. Horror is all around us. in our butchers shops, on our roads and in our newspapers. We tend to ignore it or pay scant attention, preferring to focus on the more pleasant aspects of life such as sport or tv. What you are unlikely to have contemplated (and may not particularly want to) is what happens inside a living brain as one fine situation becomes altogether another. Our world is inherently a dangerous place where horror respects no limits. It does not necessarily balance out as a good, fair or righteous place. These are false expectations. Tens of millions of living things are inevitably going to pay a terrible and disastrous price for coming into existence. For them the only answer is the terminator. Darwin noted that the apparent tranquillity of nature hides a massive slaughter from view. The majority of complex living things that come into existence – including predators - will not even attain breeding age let alone a full life. Those that get through the first hurdles are destined for a precarious and competative life. Life, death and horror are inseparable bedfellows in nature. So the facility to deal with the latter has been designed in – as standard, lying dormant in a healthy brain.

The real world – the gene world.

Human rhetoric may convince many that the world is different from what it really is. Many people have been convinced - by human rhetoric - that the world was created for mankind and that man is something completely different to all other living things. The fossil record shows something different. It shows that humans have been around for a mere fraction of the earth's existence, and a mere fraction of the history of life. (modern humans have existed for $1/36,000^{th}$ of the history of life on earth). And for only a fraction of that time has he been living in civilization. In fact for well over half of the history of life on earth the only living things were bacteria. Higher life forms such as mankind would collapse without the existance of insects but not vice versa. Humans and apes share a common ancestor – very recently in geological terms. This is not rhetoric supporting wishful thinking for a world better than the one we are stuck with. There is sound scientific evidence behind this. All that specially connects you and me is that we are of the same species, and so we can understand each other, interbreed and communicate. We have a common experience. To many this means other living things are something totally different and as expendable as garbage. My mother thinks that all crocodiles should be eradicated because they are dangerous. However she is far more likely to come to harm from her own species. As an example, 77 year old Betty Blair, a softly spoken grandmother of five from rural Texas and devout Christian was horrified at the misery in the aftermath of

Hurricane Katrina. So she opened up her home to the refugees, gave them money, clothes and food. In return within 3 weeks 3 of them had murdered her, stolen her car and $20. She was found beaten and strangled with wire in her bedroom. Mans deadliest adversary is far and away his fellow man. Contrary to the teachings of Christianity, not all people are fundamentally good. Many are fundamentally bad. It can be a big mistake to project your own good virtues into strangers. It's also a mistake to expect any help or mercy from God, irrespective of the good you do. Forever turning the other cheek is for me not the best way of dealing with the darker side of human nature. ('A criminal history of mankind' by Colin Wilson is a good summary of the evils committed by our species throughout history. Leopards don't change their spots!) Nature never intended all humans to be brothers in arms any more than starlings were designed to share food out at a bird table. We can try and make it that kind of a world but it is unlikely to last long. All species compete within themselves for the best that's on offer, and this includes mankind. Human beings are as greedy and selfish as other living things. Murder, robbery, rape, deception, fraud, street violence, slavery and war – all just part of the process of our species struggling within itself for material resources, a winning life or enhanced reproductive chances, within the confines of civilisation. Speaking of slavery, consider the massive differences in income and wealth that exist within our species. Slavery has far from been abolished. It is just more subtle. We are not united by our common humanity any more than there is a brotherhood of blackbirds. Humans are highly exploitative of each other. The rich exploit the workforce, the malingerers and feckless exploit the taxpayer. Middle aged wealthy men and attractive young women mutually exploit each other. (some of these people, functioning as prostitutes, are none the less portrayed in our newspapers as celebrities!) Of course it's so much easier to exploit people once you have conned them into the wrong mindset, as they say, 'bullshit baffles brains'. Some premier league football players aren't happy with £90,000 a week, they wants more. Meanwhile workers for Umbro in Guangzhou, South East China make £73 England shirts six days a week for a wage of £1.07 a day. They can of course top up their wages with overtime – at the princely sum of 25p an hour. When you recognise that these men who kick a bag of wind between two sticks and the average Chinese factory worker are nothing more than two members of the same species, the magnitude of the exploitative nature of human beings becomes clearer. But to many people, once someone is repeatedly in the media they seem to become a species apart, so such discrepancies become acceptable. The world has 500 billionaires who own as much as half of the rest of the world. Others are starving to death. In fact between 10 and 30 million children die every year of starvation or starvation related illnesses. It doesn't sound much like a brotherhood of man to me. And it doesn't seem to me that there is a caring creator watching over humanity – this special species the creator waited 4.5 billion years to put on the earth. Sport incidently, is our modern day substitute for the hunt. It always revolves around aiming, throwing or running. When humans first started living in civilisations they used the slaughter of animals (and people) in ampitheatres as the substitute for the excitement of the hunt. As for prey, well males will often discharge the hunting violence wired into their nervous system against each other on Friday and Saturday nights or on the football terraces. The lack of a major war has led to an unhealthy surplus of males and troublesome testosterone, so the situation is steadily becoming worse. Western societies are becoming increasingly violent. 'War..what is it good for'? asks the song. Well now I think I know. It seems a male cull is periodically required in order to maintain or re-establish stability. It's a form of eugenics, perhaps as much a part of our ecology as it is for triumphant male lions to kill the cubs of the male they have just ousted. The problem now is that we have nuclear and other weapons of mass destruction to assist in this highly repetative and possibly even necessary process.

In this world the most terrible and monstrous things can and do happen to living things on a highly regular basis. There are potentially no limits to the horror, but you can be sure that no matter what there will be no divine intervention. 300,000 men, women, children, elderly and disabled people were recently swept away by the Asian tsunami..with a total absence of any divine intervention. 1,000 people were recently killed in a religeous stampede in Iraq. Hurricane katrina recently killed thousands of Americans whilst 27 elderly people were burned to death in a coach fleeing hurricane Rita. There are no guardian angels for mice or men - or anything in between. The physical world around us is coldly and mercilessly indifferent to the plight of flesh and blood, however cruel, however unfair, however much you'd like a second chance. The only mercy and intervention you may well get when the unthinkable happens is that of your own body's defences - designed to end your life when this is the better of two bad options. I have no doubt at all that my 'depression' was the activation of this defence. Self-termination is the only possible defence available to living things in our world in the event of hopeless or horrific outcomes. What else can be done? There is nothing else. No other available form of redress exists. Near where I live in February/March on wet nights frogs and toads make an annual migration from surrounding fields to a series of ponds to breed. They cross a country lane. Though most will make it too the ponds there are always a number of individuals horribly splattered into the road by vehicles. This and countless other examples of animals mercilessly destroyed on our roads just serves as a reminder to me of life and natures subtle and inherent brutal indifference to individuals and hence why physical living things are equipped with an ultimate self terminating defence. It's also why they are designed to produce a surplus of offspring and why the number of offspring they create correlates to the magnitude of the threats they face. I believe that we subconsciously know that Hell exists, but we aren't quite sure what it is. Religion conjures up visions of fire and brimstone, a red skinned devil with horns, tail and a trident. A place where our otherwise 'all loving' God will send us for eternity just for not believing in Him. Through my illness I discovered what Hell really is. It's all the terrible things that can befall you as a physical, mortal being on our planet. And the bodies last line of defence is clinical depression – unleashing the Terminator. This process of the cruel destruction of individuals has made us what we are, different variants of a near perfect survival machine. Birds are not blinded by the sun in the same way that we are. Why? Because those that were blind to an attack coming in from the sun died out millions of years ago.

Defeat is designed in to the process.

It is statistically *inevitable* that a given percentage of all species will one way or another meet an untimely or nasty end. Nature always produces more living things than the environment can support, resulting in a struggle for existence within a species and between species. This is what has driven evolution forward. If a genetic mutation proves advantageous in the struggle for existence it inherits the earth, that's how bugs eventually develop resistance to antibiotics. It's how living things become impeccably adapted to survive their environment. At any one time lifes processes are acting as a sieve, allowing the best adapted genes to pass through and the rest to go extinct. Our bodies are made by genes which have passed through the sieve down the generations, which is why they are near optimum survival machines. Those best suited to the prevailing environmental conditions win and it's their superior genes which march forward into the next generation for the next round. In the tough competative natural world, from which we have arisen, natural selection acts on genetic variation to leave only the fittest standing. It's not a pretty picture, nor a kind one, but that's how it works. Nature consists largely a brutal war between time limited gene machines, whose only true goals are survival and replication. We are the products of a three billion year arms race. Modern human beings are part of that brutal war because they are essentially civilised stone age hunter gatherers whose numbers have exploded because of farming and medical advances. The development of a self-terminating facility is a logical and necessary inclusion for living things in our brutal and perilous world, though where it fits in with the process of natural selection I will leave for someone else to explain. The basis of the theory of natural selection is that anything which improves survival or reproductive prospects gets through the sieve. Creationists argue that some things such as the human eye and the chain of chemical reactions required for blood to clot are so complex that they could not have come about 'by chance'. Part way is no good at all. Evolutionists have shown that natural selection can in fact account for such things ie partial sight is better than no sight at all if your predators too have only partial sight. But how would they account for the existence of a terminator. How could the terminator get through the sieve? And how could a terminator not be irreducibly complex, since it is no good to be partly terminated?

The struggle for existence has driven evolution and to which we owe our very being. All living species increase their numbers exponentially beyond the limits that ecological systems can support. High wastage is expected. If other hazards don't take the numbers down then a lack of food will. Things balance themselves out as a food chain. If there are too many foxes too many rabbits are eaten. The number of new rabbits fall and so fox numbers decline, largely through infant mortality. This gives the rabbits a chance to bounce back. If there were no predators the rabbits would continue to grow exponentially and they would eventually eat themselves to starvation. Nature is the prolific creator and indifferent destroyer of life. Individuals are of little consequence. After all, one individuals demise creates more ecological space for another. So an individual life represents an opportunity with no guarantees. All living things, including humans, are ecological creatures – relying upon resources from the environment to build and maintain a physical existence. The structure of that physical existance is mostly to do with how a creature obtains it's resources from the environment. The chain of life starts from the sun with the smallest and simplest life forms using its energy to synthesise chemicals. The environment and its demands moulds living things to ecological perfection by the process of natural selection. Once a design is perfected to its environment winning becomes a case of in- fighting with ones own species, if not for food then for reproductive rights. In New Zealand an absence of large carniverous mammals allowed for the evolution of giant predatory birds to fill their ecological niche. Mammals did not begin to grow and diversify until the demise of the dinosaurs 65 million years ago, because the ecological spaces were already filled with dinosaurs. Any form of life anywhere in the universe would be recognisable to us because it would be based on carbon, that being the only element able to build complex molecules required for life. And it would be designed on the basis of what source of food it exploited. So you can instantly forget about many of our weird sci-fi monsters – they simply could never come into existance. So a fox has the perfect design to earn a living eating birds and smaller mammals. Any lesser designed animal would be driven out of existance, not just by its prey but by it's own superior peers. Far more living things of any species are born than can possibly survive, there just isn't enough food and even if there were, life's inherent and universal exponential growth of individuals would soon reach the limits of resources. If there were suddenly to be plenty for all the ensuing reproductive explosion would soon restore the norm – hunger and misery, as is already the case for many people today. Animals can't deny the drive to reproduce. But there isn't enough resources for all to survive. (though animals do find ways to restrict their numbers when their ecology is strained – typically high infant mortality.) Therefore in the natural world an individuals life is destined to be precarious and competitive. An anaconda will give birth to 25 to 100 young at a time. Given that the environment will support perhaps only one or two as adults the rest are destined to become food for camens and other creatures. It's a tough world. Exponential growth has seen to this, but without it we wouldn't have come into existence at all, because there wouldn't be evolution. Evolution enables life to find its way around natural barriers, such as the limitations of food. So we end up with creatures such as a giraffe, with a neck so long it can reach leaves out of reach to other mammals. DNA is a prolific replicator. But it isn't perfect. Mistakes are made (mutations) and in some cases these mutations confer an advantage in the prevailing environmental conditions. These genes win through to the next generation rather than their competitors. Climate change eventually alters habitats and ecosystems collapse leading to extinction for those species which have evolved to survive in a certain way. Highly specialised creatures are the most vulnerable, whilst generalists able to exploit a variety of food sources less so. (in fact, specialists are derived from the stock of generalists in times a plenty). On planet Earth one thing survives at the expense of another. As we see from any wildlife program there is no mercy afforded to nature's losers. If you're a wildebeest overpowered by lions, a colobus monkey pinned down by a group of chimps, a gazelle in the jaws of a crocodile, a gannet chick being pulled apart by two herring gulls, a mouse in the clutches of an owl, or a person whose been stood on a bus next to a suicide bomber, it's better to check out than to hang around and experience horror unlimited. Your own brain is designed not to let you. It has a terminator. So when the curtain comes down it's time to leave the stage. For each and every successful carnivore or omnivore there is an audit trail of the death and destruction of other living animals. 70% of birds nests in the UK fall foul of predation. Imagine spending 10 days on this planet and the 11th emerging from the other end of a Magpie. Not a nice outcome to your physical existence. your one and only shot at life. But these are the realities faced by living things. But your brain will never allow you to see the 11th day, because it would have already checked you out. The terminator is about serious business, it's not to be messed with. Nature is not in itself cruel, it is just callously and mercilessly indifferent to all suffering. This is why it has equipped it's living machines with a terminator. This is why clinical depression is such a terrible experience, for it is the psychology of terrible eventualities. It is the activation of a defence against horrible outcomes. Nature has seen to it that all complex living things are equipped for any life's possibilities - including the worst. This had to be the facility (mechanism) that had gone off inside my head, since my experiences could not be rationally explained by anything else. All of my symptoms and experiences pointed towards this. Morbidity, sensations from beyond the grave, horrific dreams, an affinity with death and destruction, an awesome irreversible unidirectional journey. These experiences were no coincidence. They were not the product of a low mood or spiritual illness. It all began to fit like a glove and it tied up perfectly with my observation of the merciless and prolific destruction of living things in this world. To describe or think of this illness as low spirits or a 'mood' is ridiculous and most unhelpful. It's quite simply well off the mark. I wonder if even the psychiatric world understand this illness properly. Perhaps not but I am confidant that I do.

Life is full of delusions. In our minds it is always someone or something else that is on the receiving end of the worst things in life. This is magical thinking.

Human beings are full of magical and illogical
thinking.   So many people are easy to con. After all,
we are born knowing only life and our hitherto success.
In reality everyone call meet an untimely and nasty end.
Many people have died and will continue to do so by
taking unnecessary risks, in the delusion that they were
exempt from the worst life can offer, or in the belief
that this 'good old world' will always give them a
second chance, or that God will protect them. The
world inherently takes the numbers down, it's an
inevitability. Nobody gets immunity. The rieper is a
pretty indiscriminate fellow. Nature doesn't give a jot
for individuals and God won't help either. Why have
so many people died trying to climb Mount Everest,
putting themselves unnecessarily in harms way? Why
do people drive at lethal speeds on the roads? Or do
death-defying stunts? Is it really worth the
consequences?   Having never experienced the things I
have I can see that people misjudge the consequences
and undervalue them. They misjudge the nature of life
and the magnitude of it's consequences. Having spent
so long with my life in the balance I understand and
respect my mortality. I hate speed. Speed leads to the
worst thing possible – horror. The lunatics on our
roads have no concept of it, because it hasn't happened
to them yet. It doesn't help us to understand the
consequences because from birth we are brain washed
with religious 'tribal science' indoctrination, subjected
to media mind bending, (the aquital of Michael Jackson
received many times more media attention than the
deaths of US soldiers in Iraq) fed sanitized food and

watch sanitized violence on TV. It doesn't help that most humans don't recognize themselves as just another species, having been sold the idea that the world was made for mankind who is a special case of life on earth. Religion and culture are very much responsible for these perceptions. Why did so many Japanese soldiers zealously die for their Emperor in World War II without appreciating that he was in reality just another man, just another member of the species born off an umbilical cord like every other but rather less altruistically inclined towards them. (and rather more inclined to see out his own natural life than those whose minds he has rented through ignorance and culture). Why did children in Iran use their bodies to clear minefields or become human bombs to blow up tanks whilst the man who ordered it, Ayatollah Khomeini, died of old age. It's because they are stupid and naïve enough to be taken in by the wrong reality carefully constructed by their cleverer peers who manipulate and magnify their natural inclinations to altruism – something apes also have. Super tribes make super men out of mere mortals. They do this because humans were really intended to live in small tribes of 60 to 100 where everone knew each other and their relative status. But now our tribes number millions and relations have become so deranged that some are prepared to sacrifice their one and only existance for essentially a stranger and genetic rival simply on the basis of his supertribe status. Can you envisage one blackbird blowing itself to pieces at the behest of another. They're not that stupid. They know that all of them arrived into this world in the same way and are all more or less equal. But blackbirds, having no true language, are not vulnerable to 'memes'. Memes are ideas functioning as viruses of the mind. They are passed from person to person. They take over the mind which then becomes the slavish devotee of the meme, assisting in its protection and reproduction as does a cell when it has invaded a virus. You can clearly see this in religion, legends and beliefs such as astrology, as well as cultural beliefs such as that the Emperor or Ayatollah's life is worth so much more than your own. Or in screaming hordes greeting a mere naked ape who happens to be a pop star. (In France between 1520 and 1630 there were over 30,000 werewolf trials.) You can dress someone in fancy robes, fine jewellery, endless sequins, put a crown on his head, give him a fancy title, or put him prolifically in the media, it is still just another member of our species, another naked ape, another stone age hunter gatherer living in a hugely modified environment and nothing more. In society we play games, sometimes knowingly, sometimes not so, in order to conveniently marry up our civilized lives with the gene world and pretend we are not animals. Of course there have been many greatly influential and talented people – some of these may well have in reality been psychopaths or manic depressives. Many of our 'great' historical leaders may well have simply been psychopathic. Men who have been ruthless enough to control others through a chain of physical or psychological violence or the threat of violence have been able to control civilisations and their food supplies. Thereby other mens minds are bought or sold like those of domestic animals – your survival is ensured but you have lost control of your own destiny. And you have put yourself beneath other members of the species. The rulers of early civilisations didn't waste any time in improving their reproductive prospects at the expense of their subjects. Some had over 10,000 concubines. Some had their unfortunate living concubines entombed with their dead bodies. And this bizarre, pointless and cruel act took place because of…memes. What better way to control or deter potential rivals than by steeping your worldly privilages in 'divine' rights, or selling yourself as some sort of superior entity rather than just another member of the species. But you don't have to look back in time to see vivid examples of natures selfish gene in operation in your fellow man. King Mswati III of Swaziland presides over some of the poorest people in Africa. He is about to throw a £1 million birthday party. He has ten wives, each with a palace and BMW, and 23 children. His father had 60 wives and 250 children. He abolished the constitution and banned political parties. I wonder why! Yet many of his people adore him! Why? Because he'se …well..er..the king of course! In reality he is just another man following natures golden rule – *leave as many descendants as possible*. Because he can. Or think of Emperor Bokassa I of the central African Republic who in 1977 spent one third of his poor countries wealth on his own coronation. Among his many atrocities were his alleged butchering of children at his palace. The parts he couldn't eat were fed to his four pet crocodiles. This convicted cannibal was eventually exiled, then imprisoned before he eventually returned to his family village, seventeen wives and fifty children. In fact history is full of examples of despotic men, behaving in fact exactly like an alpha male chimpanzee does, by dominating privilages and the sexual scene with violence and strategic alliances. But the chimp uses considerable less violence and cruelty than his despotic supertribal human counterparts.

Speaking of psychopaths, my experiences with someone at work drew me to the study of anti social personality disorder. Whilst most people have an empathetic mind, 2 or 3 % of all men in all cultures are psychopaths, equipped with a ruthless, manipulative and predatory mind. They have no conscience and no empathy towards others. Something is absent from their humanity. Have you ever wondered why man can do such unspeakable things to his fellow man? I would recommend anyone reading Robert Hares 'Without conscience: the disturbing world of the psychopaths amongst us'. Contrary to popular belief most psychopaths are not axe wielding madmen. There may be 50 serial killers in North America but over two million psychopaths. Most live subtley amongst us and are never going to seriously break the law. The best ones aren't even noticed. They exist as sociopaths (socialized psychopath) operating at the fringes of societies tolerance. These intra species predators are strong minded, ruthless, fearless, deceptive and manipulative. They have no conscience and no feeling towards others.   They often rise to positions of power and authority, making life a misery for those beneath them in the hierarchy. And they tend to get away with it. In organisations they can drive people to suicide. Psychopaths are often falsely charming and adept at putting on a confusing mask of normality. Forget schizophrenia and manic depression, psychopathy is by far the most destructive mental problem on the planet. Wherever there is a psychopath there is a trail of destruction – a trail of misery and blighted lives. Most people are likely to have met a psychopath without ever realising it. A famous saying is 'all that it takes for evil to triumph is that good men do nothing'. The reason is that psychopaths form 2 to 3% of all populations and given the opportunity will rise to influence and wreak havoc with their vile, self-serving, predatory and nasty personality disorder. Ironically, in some situations such as a war zone or other form of tribal strife, your unfriendly neighbourhood psychopath can actually become a 'hero', to those on his side at least. ie. Mohammed al Zarcawi.

The same delusion about the nature of mankind is going on now all over the world, with many people prepared to blow themselves to pieces in reality to satisfy another mans ideology, political agenda or hierarchical ambitions, all in the belief that they have received good council and will be going to a place of paradise. There is no real evidence for this place of paradise ….just good old mind bending human rhetoric force fed to children from an early age when their minds are at their most impressionable. Apparantly Mohammed (who took a bride aged 6) conceived of a magical afterlife to convince other men to fight and die for his causes, promising far more *worldly* pleasures, such as 72 indescribably beautiful virgins and rivers of water, milk and wine, in the next life than the majority of testosterone filled young men were likely to find in their mortal existance. If you buy into this idea, and most have no choice as it is driven into them in their vulnerable, impressionable childhood, you are ready to believe almost anything. 40,000 people in Iran recently responded to advertisements in newspapers to become suicide bombers. I believe they are being sold a pup. They are being lured into altruistic suicide and that age old practice of human sacrifice with false promises. Clerics in Iran encourage other peoples children to become martyrs – but not their own – a perfect illustration of the difference between the magical world and the gene world. Is it really Jihad or just an exercise in recruiting free mercenaries? Will Bin Laden (father of 27) be paying his soldiers a war pension if they are disabled? (Osama was the son of Mohammed Bin Laden, father of 55, husband of 22). He uses religion to recruit the services of the naive to further his own ambition and ideology. Waging war with the blood of other men is one of the oldest tricks in the book. If he is so sure of his faith he would not be hiding in a cave somewhere. He would be zealously persuing his own martyrdom and ticket to paradise. There is nothing new here. Religion has over centuries been incorporated into the vested interests of the rich and mighty to further their quest for power and influence. The crusaders used their religion to justify their slaughter of their fellow man. Islamic extremists are doing the same today. The hidden goals are population control, the persuit of an advantaged life and the subjugation of rivals. Ideology is just a cloak to conceal the persuit of advantage. The reality of life means that we can't all be winners. So the struggle will always be there. The USA is the most religious western country complete with absurd Christian snake handling cults yet it also has a huge thriving legal pornography industry complete with its own depraved oscars ceremony. Such duplicity. Popular Evangelists in the USA are often multi-millionaires. Who are they really worshipping, God almighty or the mighty dollar? My religeon taught me that it was harder for a rich man to enter the gates of Heaven than it was for a camel to pass through the eye of a needle. That hasn't stopped the evangelists becoming rich or stopped the Catholic Church from amassing uncountable wealth. The mormons are very wealthy too. Guns kill thousands every year in the USA so why aren't they banned? It's because there is lots of money to be made out of it for some people. And some make lots of money out of war. A million people were killed during the Spanish Inquisition – all supposedly in the name of God. But was it all really the persuit of mortal politics and privilage? The Catholic Church wanted to crush rival beliefs because they were a threat to its wealth and control. Isn't it really the case that Jesus was killed because he was a threat to the privilaged existance of the powerful and wealthy of his day? Between the 17th and 19th centuries Christians took 15 million African slaves to the Americas. Followers of both religions in Northern Ireland conveniently forgot the 'Thou shalt not kill' commandment when it suited their mortal goals. Our minds are very vulnerable to a rearrangement of reality. The thoughts of suicide bombers are rife with magical and therefore thoroughly illogical thinking, implanted by those who decide not to become 'martyrs' themselves. How can any free thinking rational mind conclude that an all powerful creator needs the services of mortal man to destroy Gods enemies who He happens to have created in the first place? The Aztecs slaughtered thousands to appease their Gods and devised a method for extracting the heart whilst it was still beating, this supposedly being to their Gods requirements. I wonder which crank decided this and how many people died an excruciating death because of it. 15-25,000 a year are some estimates. It was all to please their sun God Huitzilopochtli so he would keep up his daily appearance. Of course the sun was going to keep rising regardless of how many people were or were not slaughtered. To please their fertility God Xipe, a person was tied to a post and shot full of arrows, the flowing blood representing the cool spring rains. The fire God required a newly wed couple to be thrown into a fire and then before death have their beating hearts ripped out. The earth mother goddess was celebrated by skinning a young female at harvest time and for her skin to be worn by the officiating priest. Followers of Scientology believe that Human beings are an exiled race from outer space called Thetans. If they were to analyse toddlers and their natural instinct to climb they might realise that they were in fact descended from ancestors who relied on taking to the trees for protection from ground dwelling predators. And indeed early humans were predated upon by big cats. 39 members of the Higher Source cult committed suicide so as to be able to travel to heaven on a space ship that was supposed to be hiding behind the Hale Bopp comet. Meanwhile David Koresh, leader of the Branch Dividians believed he was a reincarnation of both King David and King Cyrus of Persia and had been appointed to destroy Babylon. He declared he was entitled to claim any of the females in the compound including 12 and 13 year olds, fathering at least a dozen illegitimate children before he and his followers burned to death during the Waco siege. The present leader of Iran – who apparently wants to have nuclear weapons – is a firm believer in the last of the perfect Imams who was a five year old boy who went 'invisible' in the ninth century and is waiting for the right conditions to reappear and allow Islam to dominate the world. I know that every year thousands of people go missing without a firm explanation, just as surely as I am confidant that nobody who lived in the ninth century saw the 11th let alone the 21st and that no human naked ape has ever gone invisible. He also apparently believes that Mohammed flew from Jerusalem to heaven on a winged horse to get his instructions from

God. All religeons claim the occurance of supernatural events which when believed help to hold the delusion together. A world of nonsense clearly lives alongside reality. It seems to accompany all cultures. People believe in all sorts of nonsense without a shred of real evidence. They always have. It's driven by superstition - ignorance, fear and uncertainty. Logic and rationality are suspended as mankind attempts to control that which he cannot. . In a recent case in Saudi Arabia a girls boarding school caught fire in the night but the religious police would not force open the doors in case the girls were not suitably dressed. By the time they were allowed out 13 had died. Religion relies on revelation rather than evidence, that God has revealed his plans and intentions to selected individuals. Perhaps He revealed Himself to David Koresh? Or perhaps he was just a sociopathic crank who really worshipped having control over others minds and a full and easy sex life on tap. My favorite saying is 'show me don't tell me'. For me seeing is believing. I believe that what you see in this world is what you get. If you make an ass of yourself, there will always be someone ready to ride you.

The world and life have been around an awful lot longer than mankind has. Thanks to farming and medicine human beings are currently on a typical exponential growth curve (all species multiply exponentially if the environment will support it – just two elephants, a very slow breeding species, could give rise to 19 million in 750 years). The growth curve levels off into a stationary phase when environmental resistance (limits on resources) sets in. When humans discovered farming they massively racheted up the point where environmental resistance set in. Clearly, limits on food supply is the biggest form of environmental resistance for living things. Humans (or in fact the hominid lineage of the great apes) are a species that has come about because a new ecological niche became available for us following climate and consequently habitat change in Africa. Nature abhors a vacuum . It responds with speciation events. (the splitting of one species into two) Rising mountain ranges in Africa created a rain shadow in the east. The great forests shrank and open grassland filled its place. A new environment was born. New species better equipped for this new environment evolved from old stock by a combination of mutation and natural selection acting on genetic variation – designed to exploit this new habitat. (We cannot see these changes in a lifetime, only by looking at the fossil record over millennia to see how life has adapted to new environmental conditions) In a way similar to the rise of giant birds in New Zealand an ecological opportunity for an upright-walking ape arose, so natural selection created one from ancestral apes. Man and chimpanzees diversified from a common ancestor five million years ago in the same way that polar bears diversified from grizzly's, which is why we are only 1% genetically different. As we see from the evolution of giant predatory birds in New Zealand, nature can't ignore a vacuum. Particularly over the last 10,000 years our conquest of farming and medicine has led to our pushing back the environmental resistance of the natural world, such that our numbers have grown exponentially. The only alternative is to believe that God has strangely decided in the last few thousand years to massively increase the number of souls to put to a mortal test for anything between one and a hundred years. Just eight thousand years ago there were 20,000 people living in Britain. Now there are 65 million. Following an economic boom the population of Brazil rose from 70 million to 170 million in just 30 years. Is this really the work of God or is it purely down to a type of human husbandry which may have already gone too far. Mankind eventually found the cure for diptheria, typhoid and cholera. God did nothing for us. God would let anyone with appendicitis die. Farming works on the basis that if you provide ideal conditions you can exploit the exponential growth potential of living things – in both crops and animals. Exponential population growth applies to *all* living things from bacteria to blue whales. Why wouldn't it when all life has come from the same origins. In 1859 bored colonist Thomas Austin released 24 rabbits in Australia so that he would have something to shoot at. Within 10 years the shooting of two million rabbits a year had no discernable effect on the population and a century later Australia's human population was engaged in a war with hundreds of millions of rabbits. Grey squirrels numbers are growing exponentially after being introduced to the UK, driving the reds to extinction.

Now, protected by the civilizations we have created, we are effectively farming humans – and destroying the environment in the process. The equivalent of 8,600 soccer fields worth of rain forest is destroyed in Brazil *every day*. Last century the production of food in India doubled – and so did the population. In each generation the breeding base increases of a human animal biologically programmed - like all others - to over-produce offspring in the expectation that many will die. More farming creates more people creates more farming. And instead of recognizing nature as the true creator and understanding its processes most people blindly put their faith in a mythical supernatural creator who conveniently never puts in an appearance and is unavailable for scrutiny. The 1976-1986 Iran Iraq war prompted the Iranian government to encourage people to have more children. The birth rate soared by 50% from 33 million to 50 million in 10 years. It was heading for 108 million by 2006 but a quick re-think and state contraceptive schemes have managed to restrain it to 71 million. That's 37 million lives curtailed by a change in state policy. (How does the idea that we are given our lives by God fit into this?) The human population grows by 216,000 every day, that's 78 million extra mouths to feed every year, an extra billion every 12 ½ years. This will accelerate faster because every year the breeding base of our species increases, the only thing to slow it is famine, war, disease or natural disaster. Is that the future we want? In 1798 Thomas Malthus wrote a famous essay on the principle of population, explaining that food supplies could only grow arithmetically ie 3,4,5 whilst populations increase geometrically ie 4,8,16. Therefore were it not for a shortage of food populations explode. This is what farming has done to the human population. The UN predicts 50 million refugees will be on the move within the next five years as a consequence of land degradation and desertification caused by unsustainable land use interacting with climate change and population growth. Climate change is accelerating due to the ever increasing industrialisation of China and India and Brazil chopping and burning away its rain forest. 50 million is just the start, as starving desperate people on the move spark off wars over land food and water, creating even more refugees. Ecologies will collapse and more and more species will become extinct, eventually perhaps our own. But the end won't be like turning off a light. It may involve war and starvation on a totally unprecedented scale. In Britain there are over 180,000 abortions every year and members of the Church are alarmed. But once you step out of the religeous mindset you come to realise that in a sense, in the big picture, human life is not all that sacred. Being very easy to make we can have as just about as many humans (or rabbits, or anacondas) as we want. Eventually we stand to lose far more than we will gain from a human plague. We routinely neuter cats to prevent the unfortunate sight of hordes of emaciated feral cats but find hordes of feral people acceptable. (Well of course, why not when they were put here by Gods will!!) We are heading for a world of quantity rather than quality. Nothing has ever lived on our planet and sustained an exponential growth. It has to end some how. Do we really want to see bouts of starvation that kill not millions but tens or even hundreds of millions? Do we want to live in an ever crowded and increasingly violent world? The Catholic Church incidentally is against the use of condoms in AIDS and poverty ridden Africa. 6,000 people die of AIDS in Africa every day and 10% of the population is HIV positive. Perhaps those medieval scribblings are due an update. For most of the history of the human species we existed as hunter gatherers in limited numbers. Agriculture led to the development of large communities. (and laws to prevent people acting as the natural world would dictate). The Industrial revolution raised living standards and at the same time epidemics were eradicated in many areas of the world. Population growth accelerated. It reached 1 billion around 1800. By the start of the 20th century it had reached 1.6 billion, and by the end of that same century it had reached 6.1 billion. It accelerated after World War II. 2 billion were added between 1960 and 1987. The total world population at 1800 - 1 billion - was doubled in just 27 years. Most experts expect 7 billion by 2015 and 9 billion by 2050. To believe that human beings are anything other than just another product of natural laws is to me absurd. The population of every living thing explodes when there is an unlimited food supply. There is a story from Persia which demonstrates the power of exponential growth. A peasant gave the King a marvelous chess set as a present and in return he asked only for a grain of rice for the first square, two for the second, four for the third, eight for the fourth etc. The King being no mathematician agreed and ordered that the rice be brought from storage. The 12th square required a pound of rice. Long before the 64th square every grain of rice in the kingdom had been used. And even today the entire production of rice grains in the world would not meet the requirements of the 64th square. We should be thinking about quality and not quantity. The laws of nature prescribe that you only kill for food, only eat when hungry and only reproduce in sustainable numbers. This allows other life forms to coexist. Mankind has broken these rules in such a disgraceful manner, killing for sport, killing for fashion, killing for greed or cowardly glory whilst overpopulating everywhere. Killing without a conscience because he has been taught largely by religion, indoctrination and culture that he is a species apart from these other *soulless* beasts. Do we really need a Satan when we have the human race? Mankind kills without necessity and without compassion. In Zimbabwe some people make a fortune from big game hunting. It costs 55p to kill a dove, £1,500 to blast a leopard, and £3,500 to bring down an elephant. In northern Canada you can shoot a polar bear for £18,000. Often it takes many shots for the animal to sucuum and die in agony. Hundreds of shooting farms exist in the USA where you can legally blast away an inoffensive beasts life away for a few moments 'fun'. Personally I find it obscene. When people kill other people for a few moments of excitement or sadistic fun there is outrage. Do the same to animals and it's 'normal'. In China animals are skinned alive for their fur. Cats are thrown alive into boiling water. Such are in reality acts of monstrous evil morally sponsored by religion. Even if you don't believe in God there is every reason to believe in Hell. Hell exists on a Chinese fur farm. There are personal accounts and video clips on the internet which shame humanity including live animals slowly dying with their skins torn off, animals being swung by their back legs and smashed against the ground to be left wriggling with broken backs and necks or dogs having their heads stamped into the ground. When you think of the unconditional love, trust and loyalty a dog can show to a human being you have to ask exactly who are the animals. Mankind also kills his own species in huge numbers. Human rights are a transitory concept. Man was responsible for Hiroshima, Dresden, Lockerbie, Dunblane, Beslan, September 11th and the Holocaust, so lets face the reality of the cruelty and evil which exists within our species and not go round projecting it onto a snake, a creature which kills, like all predators, because the only alternative is starvation. We don't just transform ourselves, from risen apes to fallen angels, but we often transform animals from their true identity into something they are not. We like to symbolise evil so we don't have to admit where it really comes from - the human heart.

Chimps, orangutans and gorillas could be extinct in 20 years as a consequence of the increased logging trade and trade in bushmeat – to satisfy a growing population. Nobody is in control of the human population explosion. If some more advanced species were to conquer earth and treat us the way we treat animals we would likely perceive them as evil monsters. We do this in our sci-fi films. But we are the real bad guys, doing cruel and terrible things to animals without a conscience and destroying their habitat and future as we exponentially speed our way to our own human plague. By incorrectly perceiving we are above nature we may be heading for our own demise. A massively increasing population, limited natural resources, a looming world oil shortage and weapons of mass destruction – just where will mankind be at the end of this century?. Despite mankinds intelligence he is still playing natures game little better than any other animal – maximize numbers whilst the devil may care about the consequences. It's like a doomed plague of locusts chomping down a corn field. All of the great ancient civilisations ended up destroying themselves, and their inhabitants were no less smart than ourselves – mankind has not changed genetically since the stone age. I thoroughly enjoyed reading 'the animal contract' by Desmond Morris - real issues, straight talk and not a word of nonsense. Mankinds foolish misrepresentation of himself and of other living things is expertly exposed by rational straight talk. I found 'The Human Zoo' and 'The Naked Ape' highly educational too. 'The Human Zoo' explains how we have risen from the tribal to the supertribal state and all of the implications for our animal nature and behaviour.

10,000 years ago mankind realized that you could create a continuous supply of food by pushing tubers and other plants into the ground and leaving them to grow. The crops attracted animals, some of which he was able to capture and domesticate. So the hunter-gatherer living a short and precarious life in limited numbers became a farmer and civilizations developed (together with massive individual concentrations of wealth and power, and the opportunity to get on really well in life off the backs, vulnerability and limited brains of other members of the species. Something new came into being – the stranger and the impersonal society. Human numbers began to increase as the environmental resistance was pushed back. Up until then we had been just another species in limited numbers scraping a hard living out of the natural world. Hardly something spectacularly different.

Chimpanzees have 99% of our DNA. They are more closely related to us than Indian elephants are to African elephants. (Perhaps one day someone will proclaim that Indian elephants have an array of rights that African elephant don't, or vice versa.) Dogs have 75% similar DNA. A halibut has 60% identical DNA to ours. Human and fruit fly DNA is remarkably similar – a throwback to the Cambrian explosion, that explosion of life which created all the major forms of life in the world today. This explosion in the size and complexity of life forms followed the increasing levels of oxygen in the atmosphere and the development of genes which could use it to release energy far more efficiently than anything previously. Fossil records show that humans are just another branch of the great apes, created by nature and therefore subject to it's laws, and with it it's brutal indifference. Chimps are genetically closer to humans than they are to gorillas. All three African great apes are genetically closer to humans than they are to orangutans, so put us all together and the orangutans are the odd ones out. My internal organs eyes and other bits and pieces are remarkably similar to those of a horse, a pig, a mouse a bat and a woolly mammoth. Much more similar than they are in fact different. The simple reason why is because if you go far enough back we all share a common ancestor. We are however brought up to think differently.

For me the evidence that life including mankind has evolved is compelling. The embryos of a fish, salamander, tortoise, hog, rabbit and human are almost identical at an early stage of development. The gill arches of primitive fish have been modified into jaw components in higher animals and also the 3 middle ear bones in mammals. There are many examples of homologous structures in living things. For example the fore and hind limbs of all mammals consist of the exact same bones but in different sizes and slightly different arrangements to suit the particular lifestyle. One of the best lines of evidence comes from vestigial or rudimentary structures, those body bits that have no modern purpose to the animal but were of use to its remote ancestors. Thus whales have a rudimentary pelvic girdle suggesting that they evolved from 4 legged ancestors. Some snakes such as boas and pythons have remnants of hindlimbs. In humans we have a veriform appendix, of no use to us but used by some other mammals to aid digestion. We have a faint nictitating membrane in the corner of the eye used by other land animals to wipe the eyeball clean. Frogs use this membrane as a pair of goggles when they dive. Other vestigial structures in man are a set of muscles to move the ears, a non existent tail at the base of the spine, body hair and pointed canine teeth. Vestigial structures are those which make no sense except as remnants of former ancestral states. Evidence comes from biochemistry. In the blood pigment heamoglobin the 146 long beta chain of of amino acids is identical in humans and gorillas in all but one position. Humans and pigs differ by 10 positions, humans and horses differ by 26 positions. The inescapable conclusion is that both humans and gorillas evolved from a common ancestor fairly recently in geological times. Cytochrome c is a respiratory pigment. In humans and chimps it is identical in all of it's 140 amino acid positions. In the bread mould neurospora it is different in 44 positions. The amino acid sequences of cytochrome c in different life forms differ from each other in a way which corresponds very well to the evolutionary tree as derived from more traditional morphological data. Then there are homologous structures. The wing of a bat, the paddle of a manitee, the front leg of a horse and the arm of a man all look very different, yet they match exactly bone for bone, joint for joint. All that varies are their relative sizes. Essentially the same evolutionary tree can be constructed by a number of different methods. Clues from the distribution of DNA coding and protein sequences and morphological characteristics throughout the animal and plant world together with the distribution of species on islands and continents and the distribution of fossils in space and time all point to an interconnecting branching tree of life. Evolution is only a theory, but so is gravity. Would you jump out of a plane without a parachute? No credible scientific paper challenging evolution has been put forward for over a century. I believe even the Pope agrees that life evolved. We are born into a civilized world and immediately 'socialized' and indoctrinated. Thanks to religion a line is drawn between mankind and the rest of life. We separate ourselves from the rest of the natural world and consider ourselves above nature. And because our surroundings and routines are so transformed we swallow the delusion. So if you are a scoundrel, thief, rapist, brutal terrorist, murderer or sociopath you still have a whole range of human rights. But if you are a harmless chicken your existance is worth about £2 – the price of a pint of beer. If you are a game bird you can be blown out of the sky for entertainment. If you kill a chimpanzee even as it pleads for life with an outstretched hand it is not murder, it's bushmeat. In China dogs and cats have their skin and fur torn from their bodies whilst still conscious. On Reunion Island in the Indian Ocean live dogs are impailed on hooks through the snout and then towed behind fishing boats as shark bait. Is this right? Who cares as long as it suits us? We make the rules and define the morals to suit ourselves. After all, animals can't stand up for themselves. They can't tell you that they feel pain, fear and bleed just like you do. That doesn't mean it isn't happening, just that your religious and indoctrinated mindset tells you that it isn't anything like as bad as it would be for a human being. Human rights also include the right of teenage girls to procreate and get the tax payer to keep them. And for men to be serial dads and yet do nothing to bring their offspring up. It includes the right to bring unwanted or half wanted anti social and dysfunctional children into society for everyone else to have to suffer. Now our societies are becoming increasingly violent, dangerous, anti social and overpopulated as the fatally flawed ideology of *socialism* creates a marvelous breeding opportunity for the lowliest and least responsible people. When we are sent to school we undergo a process designed to convert us from biological savage hunter gatherers into civilized adjusted supertribal citizens. It doesn't always work, so we must share our streets with dangerous, violent and anti social individuals. Religion teaches us that because animals are so inferior we need fear no guilt in maltreating or destroying them. Primitive tribal peoples often show respect to the animals they must kill to survive. Civilised man treats animals as commodities often with a cruelty, brutality and indifference of Nazis. Living cattle are transformed into burgers in minutes – by the 'children of God'. We think of Auswhitz as a symbol of a unique evil. But Auswhitz occurs every single day in our abattoirs. And as the animals are made from almost identical genes to us I doubt that in reality their experience is little if any less awful than it would be for us. Blood is blood, death is death and horror is horror. The only thing that can be said in their defence is that humans have always killed animals for food and it has never been pretty. I must also admit that domesticated animals far outnumber their wild counterparts. Jews and Muslims do not permit animals to be stunned before they are killed. Is this by the will of God or by the Satan which exists within human nature? Is it just the work of the selfish gene which operates throughout nature which says 'your life, suffering and horror are of no consequence', the very reason for which the terminator has been designed into all complex living things. Personally I can see strong similarities in the religious ritualized slaughter of animals and the activities of the Aztecs. Both are acts of selfish barbarism based on mindless superstition. Civilization in which we have spent all our lives deludes us from our biological identity and in some respects the way the world really goes round – that of exponentially multiplying living things competing within their own species for existence and reproduction and whose numbers are kept in check by limited resources, disease, predation and disaster. We are part of the same process, but nowadays thanks to farming and medicine the odds are stacked much more heavily in our favour. So what do we do about it? Well like any other living thing would, we increase our numbers exponentially.

Africa doubles it's population every 23 years, Asia every 35 years. Every ten years the population of African elephants halves. Of 500,000 blue whales humans have slaughtered all but 14,000. 95% of right whales have been destroyed. 96% of black rhinos have disappeared in the last 30 years. Humans have rendered all of New Zealands giant birds extinct. 20 acres of rain forest are lost every minute. In fact we have already destroyed half of the worlds tropical rain forest. The sixth mass extinction in the history is underway. But the cause this time is not comets or natural climate change. it is caused by the expansion and activities of humans, whose common sense and self understanding tends to be overruled by their religiously inspired delusions and their compelling reproductive hormones. Our world population of 6 ½ billion is already destroying the atmosphere and ocean ecosystems and causing global warming. 25 billion tons of CO_2 are added to the atmosphere every year. Scientific belief is that the impact of global warming over the next 100 years, somewhere between 1.4 and 5.8 degrees C, will be between severe and catastrophic. Our main response is to….increase the worlds population by another 2.5 billion over the next 45 years and greatly increase industrialization. Already 17 major oceanic fisheries are being fished beyond capacity, with nine in a state of collapse. Between 1950 and 1994 the haul of fish from the sea quadrupled. Atlantic cod breed prolifically but are still in a deep decline. It is estimated that there will be no commercial fishing left by 2048. Half a billion people face a water shortage every day. Water is going to become a big issue as countries build dams to retain it from rivers to use on their increasing need of food and industry. The countries downstream will not be amused. It takes 25 bathloads of water to produce a cotton T-shirt, 11,000 litres to produce a quarter pound beef burger and 3,000 litres to produce a kilo of rice. What are things going to be like a generation or two down the line? But then why worry when we are *magically* protected by our *sacred* status! And we know this because....well we have been told so...by other humans who lived centuries ago in a totally different world when they though the earth was flat, was only a few thousand years old, that the sun went round the earth and no one had ever heard of genes, DNA, Neanderthal Man or dinosaurs. And the world population was but a small fraction of today's. The great religious books were written not in an age of greater enlightenment, but in an age of ignorance. The passage of time doesn't alter that simple fact. They didn't know about David Koresh's of their day, the psychopaths, manic depressives and schizophrenics among them happy to spin a good yarn. The Bible puts the earth at between 3 and 7 thousand years old! The reality is that human beings are just another life form, another placental mammal, and as with other living things which temporarily overcome their natural environmental resistance our success is likely to become our downfall as, in competition with each other, we strip the world of its resources and destroy the habitat of other living things.

BACK TO THE TERMINATOR

Unlike in films where the good guys always win or die on a high note the real world often sits by without pity, intervention or the offer of a second chance for it's many unfortunate individuals. Hollywood endings are another delusional influence on our minds. As a depressed patient I felt the merciless indifference of the physical world around me. I could feel how the world around me cared absolutely nothing for the plight of flesh and blood. These are not normal healthy feelings but the fact that I experienced them as a depressed patient only points again in the direction of the true nature of my experience – the triggering of a defence appropriate in mortal defeat or terrible circumstances. And it taught me that the world offers no intervention or compassion as living things come and go. In a world in which horror knows no limits a self terminating defence may well be the only help you are going to get. Nature is callously and mercilessly indifferent to all suffering, so it's living subjects have appropriately been equipped with a terminator. The same defence facility is spread throughout the complex animal world by descent with modification, just like eyes, lungs and kidneys have. It's as essential as having an adrenaline based fight or flight system – again widely distributed throughout the animal kingdom as a survival tool. But like a hedgehog curling up in the path of an advancing juggernaut, a system, which was designed for the natural world in which it has worked so effectively for tens of millions of years, was failing me disastrously in the modern world. And I will explain how and why.

People generally don't appreciate the existence of this facility or fully understand (or wish to understand) how the world really goes round, so depression is popularly thought of as some kind of spiritual problem which the sufferer can perhaps even sort out themselves. Happiness is on one side of the coin and depression the other!   However, depression, of the type I was suffering is not about how you are feeling about life. It is not a 'mood' disorder either. It is a terrifying, disabling and extremely horrible clinical condition in which the body's ultimate defence has been accidentally brought into play. Without medical intervention it is lethal as the brain irreversibly shuts itself down. It's not simply the opposite of or absence of happiness as many people seem to think.

Mistaken beliefs.

I had grown up to believe that the only thing inside my head was me. There was the mind (which was me) and there was the body. If something went wrong with your body then you went to see the Doctor. But if something went wrong with your mind then it was 'you' and you could sort it out if you were tough enough. This was the biggest and costliest error of my life. Of course I knew there were mental hospitals and mental patients but I suppose I just thought these must be feeble people who just couldn't handle life or themselves. My mindset about depression and mental illness was deeply flawed. True I am a person and the only person in my head. But there is more inside my head than 'me'. 'I' may have been 22 years old but the genes which built the machine that I live in are hundreds of millions of years old. They are copies of genes which came into being hundreds of millions of years ago and succeeded in the red tooth and claw of the natural world with it's brutal struggle for existence. Every living thing today can trace its origins through an unbroken chain of winning ancestors who managed to reproduce before they perished. There are also unconscious, impersonal biological components inside my head which were designed for life in the natural world. They don't necessarily work in perfect harmony with the conscious personalized and specifically human parts. Having some control over my brain machine deluded me that I was in complete control of everything inside my head. Some parts of the brain simply work automatically like crude machinery in the way their genes have designed them to. Failure to appreciate this was a big part of my downfall. More specifically, the belief that all of my brain function was under the control of my conscious persona – 'me' – was fatally flawed. And it was this mistake that kept me defiantly fighting what was happening and trying to sort myself out that allowed my *clinical medical condition* to attain a colossal momentum before I eventually found qualified help. One error nearly cost me my life, but I realise now that *one error* often does in fact cost people their lives.

The brain is said to be reptilian, enveloped in a mammalian case with a human neo cortex added. The reptilian part houses the emotions (it's been suggested that is why humans can be so inhumane) and doesn't communicate with the higher more logical parts very well. I had no concept of this and no concept of clinical mental illness. I had no understanding of the inner workings of my brain. To me, aged 22, everything inside my head was me the person and I was in control. If something went wrong then it was up to me to sort it out - because I could!!! As it turned out – it was nearly the end of me! But then I suppose it's fairly normal to be naïve and gullible around aged 20. I can think of the tens of thousands who zealously signed up for their own slaughter in the First World War. (Nearly 20,000 young British men were killed on the first day of the Somme alone.) There seem to be a shortage of middle aged suicide bombers. Young people commonly make mistakes and I was just one of them. Some make even bigger mistakes than I did and pay a bigger price. A 17 year old I went right through school with decapitated himself in a motorbike accident traveling at high speed round a sharp bend. Just one of many young men speeding who every year find out too late how little the world really needs them. How their 'guardian angel' doesn't in fact give a damm. Young people view their lives and futures with rose coloured spectacles, not realising its many pitfalls and, for most it's limited opportunities. I was recently in a few pubs in Glasgow during the day and all I could see was sad defeated people in need of booze to temper their emotional pain. And young people have yet to understand fully how selfish and exploitative their fellow man can be. Who really is your enemy..is it the man in a foreign land you don't know or the man that you do who is telling you to take up arms and fight his war for him. History remembers Kings and Generals who live, not soldiers who die. If you want to get through life successfully you must recognise and take your opportunities, and where possible make them. Life shakes up people into winners and losers. It made me a loser. Many young lives go astray as their magical vision of life nurtured in childhood is derailed by the buffers of a harsh adult reality, a world of winners and losers in a zoo man has built for himself.

I would describe my depression as being inside my head but outside of me. It just came from nowhere. I didn't ask for it, I didn't cause it, want it or start it, it just happened. If only I had known that there was more to my brain than 'myself'. That my brain contained a standard lethal defence facility - entirely fitting in a world which potentially can do such terrible things to me. But that this mechanism could be triggered into action accidentally even though my life was not really in danger. That I could not stop it once it had started. Then I would have gone for medical help so much sooner instead of spending months fighting it and hopelessly trying to 'pull myself together' whilst descending further and further into a horrific and ultimately terminal illness. Unfortunately I had to find out the hard way that there is a stark difference between how you are feeling about life and clinical mental illness. I had to find out the hard way that when health breaks down there are some really serious, cruel and horrible things that can go wrong inside a normal head and that once they start you are powerless to stop them irrespective of your toughness, manliness or anything else you can summon. No man is mightier than his own mortality.

Society, general understanding and my upbringing had not prepared me. Like me there must be a lot of patients who have delayed getting help because they didn't really understand what was happening to them and tried to deal with it themselves. The public generally understand little about such illnesses. Once activated clinical depression gathers a colossal, unstoppable and terminal force, ultimately leading to stupor in which the patient sits silent and motionless.

Trying to stop it yourself is futile – it can't be done. Electric shocks may be needed to save the patients life at this stage. Friendship, money, family, love? I have experienced all of these things but they don't compare with the awesome might of clinical depression. It is the ultimate force. We know that the body has tremendously powerful survival instincts. A drowning man will clutch a piece of straw. What we don't generally know is that it also has equally awesome self terminating powers. Why did I grow up knowing about the dangers of drugs, smoking and driving too fast but not knowing anything about the terrible and uncontrollable things that could be unleashed inside my own head? I paid a terrible price for this. In some films, such as the Hellraiser films, and 'crash' (the older version where people get erotically aroused after a car crash) a link is drawn between pleasure and horror as if the two are or can be the same. In my experience pleasure and horror are as far apart as two things could possibly be. Real horror is the last thing even the most demented mind would want to experience.

Depression is almost universally thought of as some kind of spiritual problem, or an emotional issue. Medical books describe it as a 'disorder of mood' as if it is just some extension of the normal ups and downs of life – an exaggerated and protracted 'low'. Something for softies or feeble people perhaps. (though I don't doubt some people jump on the sick note bandwagon). My medical encyclopedia reads: '**depression.** In general: a disorder of mood; protracted and disproportionate melancholy'. My dictionary says: 'Affect with low spirits.' My thesaurus: depression dejection, despair, despondency, downheartedness, gloominess, hopelessness, low spirits, melancholy, sadness.' In respect of my illness these descriptions are hopelessly inadequate. A book entitled 'the body machine' is a bit better: 'In non situational depression, usually of greater severity, the persons reactions are more morbid in character; he mulls over his past, blames himself for his predicament, can see no future and may contemplate suicide. The depressive emotion is anguishing in nature and permeates all the persons thoughts and actions: actions are slowed and lethargic, it becomes difficult to concentrate or remember things, relationships and friendships become meaningless, a general running down of bodily function. People who are depressed not only look depressed, they look physically debilitated as well.' As a patient I found it intolerably frustrating that depression is thought of as a spiritual or mood problem. If everything I could wish for suddenly came to me it would not have changed me – because I was medically ill. It seemed the whole world was out of step with what was happening to me, which made things worse. On the outside I would have appeared weird, somewhat vacant, confused, quiet and withdrawn. (hardly endearing me to new friends.) Inside I was living in Hell. I felt like I was hanging on to existence by the skin of my teeth. Depression, of the type I was suffering, is poorly understood because it is the *accidental* triggering of a facility which people generally don't know is there anyway.

In summary, our bodies were forged not just from conception but over millions of years in the red tooth and claw of the natural world. A world in which the majority of things born into it will suffer an early and quite likely very unpleasant exit. A world in which horror and suffering respect no limits. A world without Doctors, hospitals, morphine, drugs or antibiotics. A world in which serious illness or injury spelt the end. Living things needed to come prepared with their own form of redress and they did this - with the terminator. If you look at the horrors on our roads, our battlefields, in our slaughterhouses and in the natural world the incorporation of the terminator into living things makes perfect sense. For this reason I know that my conclusions about my illness must be right.

Civilisation only began 8-10,000 years ago. Whilst it steadily improved our chances of survival it also brought unnatural stresses and pressures that we were not designed for. If stresses and anxieties combine sufficiently at a vulnerable time they can become indistinguishable to the unconscious primitive parts of the brain from an imminent disaster, giving rise to the unleashing of the terminator. Therefore leaving a confused and bewildered person unknowingly heading for the end of their life. This is the true face of clinical depression – the unleashing of the terminator.

Design limitations and the problem of modern life.

There was no threat to my life, no imminent disaster. But there was a lot of stress, nervous ill health and anxiety. This was the precursor. Evolutionists say that the human brain evolved to meet the demands of the African Savanna where we originated. Only real life threats could produce severe or prolonged anxiety in such an environment. But the unnatural stresses of modern life in our concrete world can combine to produce severe and unnatural levels of anxiety. (Suicide is the biggest cause of death in 16 to 24 year olds). Loneliness, social isolation and exclusion, heartbreak and work related stress can combine to produce something that our unconscious 'natural world' brains were never designed for. Eventually something has to give. Designed for the natural world we are much more fragile mentally than some of the *combinations* of pressure, stress, frustration and anxiety that modern life can throw at us. We have a design specification intended for a life in the natural world – that of a stone age hunter gatherer. Go beyond it and we are in trouble. But our modern world can easily do just this. This makes clinical depression a statistical inevitability for a given percentage of people living in the pressure cooker modern world. The psychiatric people are ready in waiting for the casualties, of which there would be far fewer if understanding about these illnesses were brought into the public domain. We are a branch of the great apes designed for a precarious and hard but mentally free hunter-gatherer existence. But we are living in an overpopulated, concrete, highly technological, spiritually sacrificial, antisocial, economically unfair rat race. It favours our physical survival but not necessarily our happiness and mental well being. Get on the wrong side of it and you could be in trouble. We don't live in small communities where we all 'belong'. We live in a greedy, unfair, mentally manipulative, exploitative, overcrowded, media mind bending, selfish and often impersonal supertribe where individuals can easily become marginalised, isolated or left on the scrap heap. We can largely thank a supertribe society based on money for this. Humans were made to co-operate, not go it alone, so social isolation – a common problem in the impersonal supertribe - leads to negative and destructive stress. In individuals such as Thomas Hamilton of Dunblane it can explode into a terrible vengeful rage. Our society, a supertribe of small nuclear families surviving off money literally creates isolated unwanted nobodies out of many of it's citizens. It's little wonder life can get confusing or that there are so many problems. We have built a world that greatly favours our physical survival, but we pay a mental price for being out of our natural environment and not living our lives as nature intended. How many people are stressed, lonely, mentally ill or have anxiety disorders – quite a lot. How many people resort to drugs or alcohol every day to achieve a false dawn? It's no wonder we get stressed having to interact with so many people who we do not know and potentially could do unto us psychological or physical harm. Like monkeys and apes we have the skill of looking into anothers mind to predict what we are likely to get from them. But to do this reliably takes time. You can't do that with everyone you meet in a supertribe. It's fertile ground for liars, sociopaths and con men. Drugs, alcohol, smoking, violence, suicide and mental illness are all a consequence of our lives in our unnatural concrete jungle. Those who succumb to the stresses and pressures that accompany social marginalisation or can't adjust to earning a living in an unnatural way become our weirdoes, bums, dropouts and tramps. They have been overtaken by anxiety, a common, disabling and easy to aquire illness. By staying in my stressful environment whilst suffering a reactive anxiety state I had entered into an escalating spiral of stress, anxiety and ill health. This was a very vulnerable time for me. I stayed in the firing line, brave, noble but naïve and stupid – just like the First World War volunteers and Irans boy soldiers. My life had become unhealthily empty and without my friends I lost the ability to release some of my 'working life' frustrations at weekend. I had fallen into social exclusion – a common pitfall for modern humans. This happens because of the way our societies have been constructed. We don't live in tribes, but in greedy self centered supertribes. Social exclusion in itself is an unnatural state for human beings and leads to a deterioration of mental health. Suzanne broke my heart; I had become extremely fond of her. Did I deserve it? Not really. Losing our dog and my friends completed the emptiness. My supportive network had fallen apart – a common fate awaiting people who cannot keep up with change or build a wide and strong enough network, or make all the right moves. And it had happened at the worst possible time, when my work pressures were escalating. The consequence was a reactive anxiety state. Pressure and stress at work turned this anxiety into an escalating spiral. When I transcended my natural limits – those set for a life in the natural world - the 'terminator' came into play. This was an inevitable consequence of the way I have been designed – a stone age hunter gatherer living an unnatural life in a modern concrete jungle.

Having only a small and narrow supportive network was one of my failings. You could say my anxiety mimicked an imminent disaster or that I simply went over the threshold for anxiety and incurred the inevitable next step. Either way it is clear that our brains are not designed to accommodate continually escalating stress and anxiety. And they are unable to discriminate one anxiety from another. The relationship is simply stimulus and response. These are the brains design limitations. If you suffer severe anxiety – regardless of the cause – your unconscious primitive brain treats it as imminent disaster, *because it has been designed that way*. It has been designed for life in the natural world. 'The anxiety comes first..then the depression' as Dr. Callan commented. Depression is the end game of escalating anxiety. But it is the *nature* of the 'depression ' that I found to be poorly understood. Most people understand depression as low spirits. Real depression is much more serious and awful than that. It is highly ruinous, true clinical illness. It is horrific and lethal. And for many it is the end of their lives.

Darwin noted that body parts such as limbs and wings were often not perfectly designed for their roles but were simply nature doing the best with what it already had to start with. The frontal fins of bony fishes have become turned into fore legs, arms, wings and flippers. The human brain is the same. It isn't a perfect device, in so far as it is just the best nature could do with what it already had to work with, a modification to what has gone previously. A more advanced brain has been built on top of a cruder more primitive one. In a similar vein the human eye is far from perfect. It has a blind spot, easily detachable retina and its sensory receptors face the wrong way so we have to process diffuse light. Why does it have these failings? Why did 'God' give us an imperfect eye? It's because the vertebrate eye was derived from the eyespot of the humble lancelet – a sand burrowing filter feeder.

The brains primitive internal systems – designed for the natural world, can be easily fooled. Consider pornography. Pornography (for many a surrogate sex life) doesn't exist in the natural world. But celluloid or magazine pictures can arouse the body's reproductive systems as if a real sexual opportunity is imminent – which it generally isn't. The adrenaline fight or flight system can be evoked simply by watching a scary movie, making a speech or sitting an exam. It isn't really required – we are not confronting a lion or a crocodile. The point is, we were made for a life in the natural world and derived from living things that have been living in the natural world for hundreds of millions of years so the brains inner workings cannot make the distinctions. In the same way severe anxiety 'fools' the brain into acting as if terrible things are imminent. I know I am not about to have sex when watching pornography and I know that I am not about to be eaten by lions when suffering anxiety related to an unfortunate turn of events. But try telling that to the primitive unconscious – designed and programmed over hundreds of millions of years for the natural world – a world in which existance is inherently brutal, short lived, nasty and precarious. In the natural world, for which we have been designed, sexual arousal means mating opportunity, adrenaline situations means flight or fight and severe anxiety means imminent unavoidable disaster. As much as I suffered I don't begrudge my terminator, because I understand why it is there. It is there to spare me from excessive suffering. It is an ally in a dangerous mortal world. I only wish it was more sophisticated...but it isn't. It can be brought into play when your life isn't really in mortal danger. And I wished I had known about it before it struck. Lack of understanding meant my illness reached a colossal magnitude before I obtained treatment.

When anxiety exceeds our design specification the defence is triggered, regardless of whether our lives are really in peril or not. Primitive internal systems can't make a distinction between 'modern day' anxiety problems and mortal disaster. Once activated the defence is awesome and unstoppable as it is fundamentally beyond voluntary control. Irrespective of my level of courage and resilience I needed the intervention of psychiatric medicine to save my life. I'm not ashamed of it. If there is any shame it belongs to society for not educating people about such things. How was I to know what was happening to me? Surely it's better to educate people about mental illness than to wait until people are horribly ill and then crudely try to deal with the consequences.

What next?

And so here I was, in a living hell. I thought about suicide very regularly. I was in the world of the undead, dead and alive at the same time. A terrifying, devastating and highly undesirable place to be. (it does you no good to spend a lot of time here - it eventually breaks your mind and destroys your soul) But I was brave, intelligent and fundamentally a good person. I would go behiend the bird aviary at home clench my fist and scream inside at myself 'Im going to win, I'm going to win, two more months and you will be ok, just two more months. You can take it for two more months'. When I was growing up my older brother would bully me but whenever he hit me he would always get one back, even if I came off worst. At school I had fights with guys who were bigger than me. But I would win by taking the punishment and outlasting them. I was deceptively tough and this has caught out many people. In my teens I was very much into boxing and martial arts. I was I believe a natural fighting man..and reasonably intelligent with it. Intelligence, fighting instincts, self love and being fundamentally a righteous and good person were the weapons with which I stood up to the terrible daily punishment on the terrifying edge of eternity. They were the weapons with which I confronted the decision..'do I give up on living in this seemingly terrifying, futile and pointless world or take the terrible punishment and carry on'. At these crossroads many opt for suicide. They 'take their lives while the balance

of their mind is disturbed'. What was to be the
outcome for me?

Two illnesses for the price of one.

The months rolled on and things didn't seem to be getting much better. In some ways I was more afraid of my future going to ruin than what was happening to me now. I tried hard to present myself as normal. I did go for some pub lunches with Suzanne but she was still with her boyfriend. In fact I concluded that she was living with him and I was right. That upset me. It probably made me feel even more isolated. I never said what was wrong although it must have been obvious something was. I thought this may be detrimental to any future prospects with her. I studied A 'level human biology. I read everything five times but it soon disappeared from my mind. Our central office at Newcastle went on long term strike. Our local office manager wouldn't allow overtime. I was working flat out for 10 hours a day. I noticed new symptoms, such as teeth grinding and music in my head which I had difficulty in switching off. I believe that I was starting to suffer from mental breakdown, neurosis and psychological degeneration. The psychologist, who I had seen a number of times, and who's only contribution was to provide me with a relaxation tape and technique (involving alternately tensing and relaxing my muscles in bed) suggested that I was well past the time when medication was effective and that she was sure that Dr. Callan wanted to take me off it. I felt terrified, for I felt that if I was left in the state that I was currently in I would be compelled to eventually commit suicide. I was getting desperate and frustrated with my progress. I asked my GP for more medication. 'Lets see how you get on' he said. I felt like ringing the Samaritans. I no longer felt that I was being handled by caring or even competent people. I didn't feel like a valued member of society any more, a normal person with an illness. I began to feel that I was just unimportant psychiatric scum without rights, say or self-determination. The psychiatric people just didn't seem to care enough, and I began to feel that I wasn't in especially competent hands. But they were in total control. Looking back I suppose I was secretly starting to realise that my prospects of making a successful and healthy recovery were fading – and there was no one to help me. I was descending into a long term secondary illness. These professional carers, who held the key to my future, to me were just not good enough and there was nothing I could do about it.

After two years of treatment I was on the verge of going to University to study Ophthalmic Optics. I approached my GP for more help. I saw a locum – Dr. Coaker four times. Dr. Coaker sniggered to himself when I told him that I thought I knew what was wrong with me and the people who were treating me didn't. He referred me to a psychiatric nurse who suggested some sort of injected medication. I didn't have any confidence in his competence. My perception was that he didn't see me as a sick person who was desperate to live a normal life again, but that I was just another lost cause to give a new type of drugs to on an endless treadmill. Dr. Coaker said that he didn't want to change my medication without Dr. Callans approval. He promised me a referral to Dr. Callan. I waited, but nothing came. I found out many years later that Dr. Coaker wrote in my medical records that he felt sure that I would be unable to cope with the demands of University. I wrote to the University medical centre to tell them that I was ill but I never heard from them.

So I left my job in the Civil Service after seven and a half years and started University. It was tough. Living in a fog didn't help. The math's was way over my head and I felt more socially isolated despite meeting new people. But I tried very hard. My mother paid for me to have private maths tuition. There was a Civil Service function which I went to. Suzanne was there. She told me that she was splitting up from her boyfriend. I asked her out and she said yes. I felt upbeat about that. But a week later I got a letter from her saying they were not now splitting up and she was apologetic but couldn't do what she had promised. I wrote back telling her how upset I was. That Christmas I had a good kissing session with her at her office but her boyfriend then came and picked her up. I was getting increasingly stressed with my course. Coming up to my final exams I began running long distances to relax my nerves. Half way through my final exams I had a breakdown. I couldn't get up. My head and nerves were going crazy. I phoned my mum and she was mortified. I was interviewed by two tutors. Neither had the slightest empathy or comprehension of what I had been going through. Nothing new there.

My own tutor – a Ph.D., said almost in disbelief 'well now is the time you should be enjoying life, the problems come later with the responsibilities.' A very intelligent man no doubt but like most people clearly unable to understand the difference between a healthy person with a few problems and one with the effects and consequences of a clinical mental illness. This highly educated man had no more understanding of mental illness than I had on my 20th birthday.

Term over. I returned home and saw my GP. I told him I thought I had manic depression as I was suffering alternating bouts of elation and being down. My nerves and my mind were out of control. I asked for a referral to Dr. Callan. 'Oh it's just you' he angrily said, 'you've been on the stuff for a year…more!' He had clearly lost his patience. In truth I was in a state of disablement and savage ruin. I had been through three years of terrible punishment. I had desperately tried everything in my power to protect my future and regain my health. And I had failed or as I genuinely believed and still do, the NHS – and society - had failed me.

Broken man, broken mind, broken future.

And so here I was, after three years of treatment for depression by the NHS. A broken and savagely ruined man. Without a soul, without an identity. Lost in a fog. Broken life, broken mind, broken man, broken future. Lonely and unemployed. Suffering from anxiety, neurosis, mental breakdown, alternating elation and depression, the effects of long-term depression and long term drug use, in chronic pain and discomfort, my nerves completely out of control. But there was more. I felt like I was in the gutter – forever, there was absolutely no trace of a route to normality. Mental illness destroys identity and the meaning of and quality of life. Have you ever wondered what it is like to lose your soul? I can tell you. After three years of treatment and trying so hard and with such bravery and resiliance I had been left with a complex unbeatable and untreatable disability. And so I should say that at this point I was for all practical purposes ruined for life. There was no route to recovery or normality. When things go wrong your own nerves can lock you in an unbearable and inescapable prison which you can never really understand unless you have been there. So as always, nobody understood. And I firmly blamed the people who had treated me because I had developed a very strong belief that I had been under diagnosed and given treatment which was inadequately effective. I had been returned to the same stressful working environment which had contributed much to my illness in the first place, out on my feet and experiencing horrific suffering - with just a low dose of anti depressant. And all in the belief that all Doctors were caring and competent people, that I was in good hands and would get right again in a few months. I could easily have killed myself. It's not down to the psychiatric people that it didn't happen. And it wasn't down to God either. My prayers went unanswered as I suffered a misfortune I largely didn't deserve. It was down to *my* courage, *my* resilience. I survived the terminator but I was effectively left disabled and destroyed. They say God helps those who help themselves. Well I helped myself and now I don't feel the need for God for anything. (However to quote a World War 2 submariner: 'when you are down there silently waiting for the depth charges to go off, believe me, everyone has a God'. I believe him.)

Whilst I was slowly recovering from the original illness I believe I had been developing a secondary illness – neurosis, mental breakdown, psychological and spiritual degeneration, chronic stress cycles, largely as a consequence of prolonged appalling suffering. I was accumulating long term psychosomatic damage. Not a clinical mental illness but perhaps something more akin to shell shock – the system getting unhealthily rearranged by going through far too much. This is known as a functional illness. The generation of the secondary illness was indistinguishable from recovery from the first. Under the circumstances I feel that this was the rather inevitable consequence of the failings in the treatment and care prescribed to me by the NHS. Neurosis, mental breakdown and the deterioration and submission of my mind and will had overtaken the relief from the original illness. One illness had led to another – I was deeply ruined and destroyed individual left, after 3 years of punishment, with many mountains to climb. And without good support, good treatment or understanding it's easy to see why some people take their own lives, or spend the rest of their days defeated and living in squalor.

I eventually protested my way to an appointment with Dr. Callan. I noticed his hands shaking. I wrote down all my symptoms. He tried to be calming. 'There's nothing seriously wrong with you' he said. I think he should have clarified the situation better, maybe something like 'you do not have a psychotic illness, however you are at the very least semi – disabled, your identity has been all but erased and you have mental breakdown and neurosis which is untreatable and will at best take years to outlive, other than that there's nothing seriously wrong with you - now please get on with life. After all you are just a poor confused psychiatric patient and I am a qualified consultant with lots of qualified friends and colleagues so how will you ever be able to demonstrate that I have botched your treatment?' As before he was master of the understatement. I believe he knew he'd messed it up and was secretly filled with guilt and embarrassment. He did say that he didn't want to put me on pills for my out of control nerves because I would end up on them for the rest of my life, and I could understand that. Looking back I should say that I had a cocktail illness, a painful and intolerable mental prison with no key to the door. To this day I blame this largely on a poor and sloppy diagnosis, followed by inadequate medical treatment, support and care, from whom I came to consider as cold and incompetent people. I survived, but I believe this was only because I was tough, brave, a good person and because I had the intelligence to understand something of what had happened to me. As a natural fighting man it was in my nature to be able to absorb enormous punishment and to keep going even when beaten. (the same stupid fighting instinct which kept me trying to beat it myself for so long) Other patients don't survive. This comes as no surprise at all to me. I estimate I contemplated suicide a hundred times. This is the scariest bit – I don't believe the majority of people would have survived my experiences and I had I not been in my 20's with most of my life still left I don't think I would have either.

I saw another psychiatrist Dr. Alitt. My interview with her was acrimonious. She said that I was 'just a confused and frightened little boy' and it was 'awful how I was in a straight jacket bottling up my feelings'. We discussed my upbringing, which I found to be totally irrelevant to the present predicament. To me she talked complete claptrap. Looking back, I think she was strategically trying to shift the blame for my situation on myself and away from those charged with my care. She rubbished my opinion of my illness saying 'that only happens to old people' and said that my depression was 'grief'. She offered me psychotherapy involving holding hands with other patients and being led blindfolded and other seeming nonsense. I desperately wanted help, but not to be patronized as some kind of weakling or freak. I declined. The interview endeared me even less to the psychiatric profession - and I don't think I am either unfair or a fool. I thought her rhetoric was a disgraceful way for a well paid health care professional to treat a desperate, lost and sick man. As I look around I see a lot of mental wreckage. The world isn't just a physically dangerous place. Life can leave you broken minded and ruined with no way out. It's another statistical inevitability. To some they are just lazy bums. To me many are likely to be hopeless tormented anxiety state prisoners on the wrong side of life in a mean and selfish world. I believe most people who have been left truly mentally ruined will stay that way. It can be almost impossible to turn around a broken life and a broken mind. A bar customer of mine with a very good job called Eddie went on the booze after his wife died. He started to latch on to everyone for company including people with drug problems and a MENCAP group. But he became a danger to himself on the premises and began to smell revolting so I had to bar him. I still see him wandering the streets, scruffy lost and pissed. I don't think he will ever escape his prison. An anxiety disorder can be a life sentence. Society won't help. Society is largely selfish, all have limited energy and nobody wants a monkey on their back.

Many such people have no doubt been processed by the psychiatric service and left on the scrap heap. When I was 19 I worked for a few days on a ward for severely handicapped people. Some had nasty scars and a nurse explained that in the case of these patients surgeons didn't try their best when stitching up wounds. In other words, Doctors are prepared to ease off when there is less likelihood of consequences. I think a similar thing may happen in psychiatry. Perhaps it wasn't the best decision to have my first psychiatric appointment alone. I'll never really know.

Around 13% of adults in the USA have an anxiety disorder. These are illnesses, not personal weaknesses, but personal weaknesses will tend to creep in when a disruptive or painful anxiety related problem cannot be overcome. When people say someone has a 'drink' problem or is a drug addict they are probably really describing a persons attempt to find relief from a persistent anxiety problem or illness. People can get trapped in a cycle of stress, anxiety, fatigue, depression and sleep problems when some of the ingredients for mental health are absent or things in their life have gone wrong. I believe schools would be better spending more time teaching pupils life skills and warning them about life's pitfalls than forcing them to regularly regurgitate repetitive religious rhetoric. I would suggest that the reason religion is so repetitive is that this inhibits the mind from exploring alternative theories about life. Books such as the Bible and the Koran will contain a religious interpretation of all lifes potential twists and turns. This helps to prevent your mind from ever exploring a different reality. Unquestioned faith is considered a virtue but I believe it is the stuff of the gullible. The domestication of an elephant is achieved by putting it into a cage and subjecting it to a bullying trainer and a nice trainer. It eventually bonds with the nice trainer and it's mind is thereby conquered. Clever stuff. The creators of our religions learned how to conquer the human mind. Exploit natural ignorance, vulnerability and uncertainty and induce fear for detractors (an eternity of burning in Hell) whilst giving fabulous promises to those who comply. (An eternal life in Heaven, reunion with loved ones). Then you can introduce magical supernatural events and convince people they actually happened that way by utilising the passage of time. When I see someone aged around 60 belching out the word of God to passers by at a market square I realise religion is a powerful tool, and appreciate my free thinking mind even more. This mans mind isn't free, it is serving a virus caught from another man.

I returned to University in the summer and finished my exams. This was very, very traumatic and difficult. In the end I came sixth in my year. But I decided that I wanted to take a year out to try and sort myself out – without the help of the psychiatric profession. My GP gave me a medical certificate stating 'mental illness' and asked me how I would get by for money. Of course I could have taken the incapacity benefits route to a wasted future but I was defiant about my condition,

I wasn't going to give up on life or myself - and I elected to register as unemployed instead. I saw a student's doctor in Manchester, Dr. Lobjoit. She took a tough stance – too tough. She encouraged me to come off anti depressants and I did. She told me I must get back on my course or start another. But I didn't know what to do. What Dr. Lobjoit never really got her head round was that I was in a state of disability, lonely, highly vulnerable and not up to the demands life places on healthy people, and she had no sympathetic understanding of the terrible suffering that I had been through. Given the choice I would probably prefer to live through Aushwitz than live through severe depression. I'm not trying to demean the experiences of people who survived concentration camps, only to emphasize that my experience was also a matter of life and death and of terrible suffering. I spent more than two years holding the reapers hand - a terrible, terrible experience. So when we eventually parted company, (with herself, I assume, in a state of frustration) she did not stay on my Christmas card list. The solution was beyond her as it was beyond me, because there wasn't one.

It was decision time. I had no plan for the future but the decision was made without me seemingly making one. I was not going back to university. When I told my GP his tone lowered and I think that perhaps the penny finally dropped that I wasn't some sort of softy but a truly damaged individual. His wife, also a GP described me as 'not without intelligence'. (*Cheers.*)

She said to me 'come on just think about those soldiers who were taken prisoner in World War II. Those boys never knew if they were going to get out of it alive'. I said back in the tone of someone mentally retarded, 'oh I think I have been through something as bad as that'. 'Well ok, but now it's time to get back into the rough and tumble'. Just like that! It's easy and straight forward when it's not you. I was in a wicked trap – with both a disruptive disability with seemingly no way out yet needing to get going to try to save my future. Basically I was fucked. I wanted to claim medical negligence but I didn't know how and I was too afraid. I had never heard of a similar case. I concentrated on 'getting better'. My parents were morally useless. They had no concept or understanding of what had gone wrong or what I was now up against. But they did keep me.

Going round in hopeless circles.

The year rolled on and so did the desperate efforts to find 'normality' – a state of health, happiness and identity. I took to early morning swimming, weight training, herbal tranquilizers, long distance running, doing math's till two in the morning, and of course drinking. I even started walking all night and was stopped at 4am by the police once ten miles from home. They were stunned. I was just so desperate to find a 'cure' and a route to a decent life and to end my pain. I could spend ten minutes just deciding whether to go to the loo or not. I had neurosis. I was in a painful prison which I desperately wanted to get out of but essentially couldn't. I just went round in circles. I read books by a Dr. Claire Weeks.'self help for your nerves', 'more help for your nerves'. I realised that I was far from alone in my problems. Many people described in her books had been nervously ill for decades. She says that at the heart of nervous illness is anxiety disorder and I would agree. Dr. Weeks 'time out' tactics were of help (resting during the day) and it was encouraging to finally encounter someone who really did know their stuff. When I was in the Civil Service I worked with a man called Peter who was middle aged, divorced and pretty fragile. If his nerves got the better of him he had to go and have a lie down. Another person with a life long sentence of anxiety disorder. Such people tend to be single and isolated. Looking back, I think the best thing for me at this time would have been occupational therapy and counseling, but counseling from people like Dr. Weeks, not hard-faced patronisers like Dr. Allitt. I needed competence and I needed empathy… and I just couldn't seem to find either in the NHS.

So what was I going to do now? I didn't know and although (crucially) in a protective environment I was essentially no better than nine months ago. My thoughts went to down and outs. Many of them must be mental prisoners too, people with damaged and tormented minds with no way out, just the temporary relief of alcohol. In my life I have come across many people, mostly men, who society would look upon with disgust when in reality they are genuinely incapacitated – hopelessly and for all practical purposes permanently diseased by that most unfashionable medical condition anxiety illness. Many 'respectable' invalids probably have a better quality of life than these people do. But as Mr. Average might say..'pull yourself together' or perhaps 'they have *chosen* to live that way'. I've seen men fall from normality and respectability into being down and out, and I've met a number of people who have anxiety disorders as a lifelong problem. In the 'Lethal Weapon' films Mel Gibson is portraying a character with an anxiety disorder. It's deemed comical but I can assure you there is nothing funny about living with an anxiety illness, every day is an unpleasant experience. I was fortunate to at least have a roof over my head. At least I had a platform to try. Without that I doubt I would have ever found a way out of my impossible prison. I may well have ended up just another permanently ruined and broken (and misunderstood) man living a desperate, heartless, degenerative and wasteful life of squalor. Mentally broken people, people diseased with anxiety, need specialized help – and it isn't available, so they have to live out their days in a state of mental ruin. Society just doesn't care enough. One day my dad came home in a violent mood and threw a punch at me. I blocked it and hit him back and flattened him. He told me to leave home. There was real strife in our house at that time. I was looking at my future down the barrel of a gun. My future was potentially going to become one of permanent despair and degradation. He didn't understand my problems and how desperate I was to protect myself. A week later we were quietly doing jobs together.

Forward with uncertainty.

After several more months of going round in circles a friend who ran a club offered me a job behiend his bar. As with everything I agonised over and over but I had done bar work before and I decided to give it a go. I enjoyed it. It was therapeutic to be doing something constructive and it drew my attention away from myself. It was an important step for me. I could have gone on forever as I was but it did take courage to break free. There were challenges. Two nasty committee members made fun of me. But I let it go over my head. Eight months later I joined onto a HND in Hospitality Management. No really strong sense of direction or certainty of what I was doing. I told the enrollment tutor what had happened to me and she was understanding. She said that I had been unlucky and I really appreciated that. Empathy at last! It's a pity I couldn't find any in the people charged with my care. It was a bit of a come down to have grade 'A' A levels and have been on a degree course to be doing a HND with younger and less academically skilled people. But I was after all one of life's losers. I really wanted a route back into work and my course had an industrial year after nine months. I was ridiculed and mimicked by some students because I sounded like I was mentally handicapped – five years after Dr. Callan had told me he would 'get rid of my depression easily enough'. I think word got round that I was fighting the after effects of mental illness and I seemed to become something of a hero, they cheered me when I walked into the lecture theatre (always late), although I never discussed my past with anyone. Except a cookery teacher who it turned out had had a nervous breakdown herself and understood my plight. She criticised my sloppy food presentation and I said 'what does it matter, I'd eat it'. 'But you are doing this for customers and it is important to them, they are paying money' she explained. I knew what she meant, but at the time having been through such suffering and having had my life so horribly and terrifyingly in the balance for so long it also seemed pathetic that such things were of any consequence to anyone. My law tutor also had nervous problems, perhaps some kind of anxiety disorder. I didn't like some aspects of my course but I stuck at it.

Maybe things were getting a bit better but I was still a highly stressed, nervously ill and unhappy person. I made some friends at college. When my industrial year came I hated it. I tried to change my course and to get into leisure but I failed. I worked in an A la Carte restaurant doing split shifts, cycling to and from work 6 miles twice daily. There were problems and complications along the way but I got through nine and a half months before going to do Camp America with two girls from college. On camp I was ridiculed once or twice by campers and colleagues as a 'downer' and 'dork'. An arrogant American guy gave me all sorts of problems until I indicated to him the option of a fight. Some people just have to take you to the limit before they back off. As a person who prefers a quiet life I hate them. Six years on and I was still visibly recovering from mental illness. When I came back from the USA I returned to college for my final year. I also started working as a lifeguard at a local leisure centre and this proved to be a good move. The place was laid back, easy and sociable. I made new friends. I was still worried about my future – it seemed no potential job or career could make me happy and I felt the opportunity for marriage was passing me by. Why couldn't I just meet 'Miss Right'? I now know why. There has not been a major war for 60 years and so society has excessive males. Wars are a male cull and serve to rid the species of excessive troublesome testosterone. Calm eventually returns and those males remaining have enhanced reproductive prospects. 24% of the male breeding population in Britain were killed in the First World War. Interestingly, in societies where there is no formal system of punishment, males kill 25% of other males. Combine this lack of war with an epidemic of single mothers and a confused and stressed man in his late 20's/early 30's is really up against it.

The late graduate.

After my HND I went to upgrade to a B.Sc. at Manchester. It was so much harder than the HND. The other students were so clicky; in fact they were down right horrible. I thought I would have a good time in a class which was almost all young girls, many of them attractive. I was wrong. A lot of girls aren't nice at all to men for no seemingly good reason – God knows what they are reading. Perhaps they hate the filthy desires and polygamous sex drive all men possess. I'm afraid it comes with the species. And many men – like me – can handle it and show respect even if we can't change the way we have been made. Most of them marginalised me. I felt so lonely, desperately lonely. I nearly packed it in. My loneliness was crippling. I went to the pub at night on my own and stood there like a jerk watching everyone else in groups having conversation – not the nicest experience. At least I got to go home at weekends where I was able to work at the leisure centre. The final exams came. I was completely stressed out, we all were. On my first exam I must have had an adrenaline dump or panic attack because I froze for ten minutes. But I took them and I got a 2i BSc. (HONS). When I left University I felt a decisive lift. Maybe with constant home and leisure centre and new friends I had finally achieved a good level of stability. But what was I going to do job wise? I was only a casual. I worked for two years doing a variety of casual jobs. I didn't want to work in hotels or restaurants as they had a reputation for long hours, low wages and exploitation. Eventually I got a job in management. I was still stressed, still neurotic, still anxious, but I started to feel at long last that I might have been eventually able to find a normal, happy and healthy future.

As for Suzanne, she married a policeman. I stayed in touch until the last three years but I finally lost my patience because she never made any effort to keep in touch with me. She visited the leisure centre twice to go swimming and I asked her to come and see me afterwards but she didn't. I was really deflated about that. It would have been so much easier to have given up all those years ago and been a bum but here I was, a graduate holding down a Management job and she couldn't be bothered to see me! I never told her what was wrong. She must have worked out that I had some sort of Depression but would never understand what had actually gone wrong. But I think she was romantically cruel to me. I also felt she had not been sympathetic enough and was letting me down as a friend. Suzanne seemed to look down her nose at me, she left me high and dry when it suited her and I eventually left her to it. Suzanne had seemed my dream girl, so nice, so fun loving. She seemed to change into being selfish and materialistic. Perhaps the DHSS did that to her. But I did learn from her, very painfully, how cruel and selfish a girl can be to a mans heart. I think it is unfair to encourage someone to like you and then pull the plug on them and never give them another chance. My anxiety state wasn't just about

Suzanne. A succession of unfortunate events had put me on the wrong and unhealthy side of life. My advice to young people who haven't many friends would be to get involved in clubs and interest groups, because life's twists and turns can pull the rug out from under your feet. Things change and situations move on, so you should develop many options and try not to burn your bridges. Relying on one or two social contacts is a dangerous game.

Is there any justice?

A few years after graduating I made a fumbling effort
to complain about medical negligence. Eventually I
found more appropriate channels. My complaint was
that I had received inadequate medication and
inadequate care as a result of Dr. Callan misdiagnosing
the severity of my illness. I said that the consequences
of this were that I was left ruined and disabled after
three years of treatment. It first went to my NHS Trust
and a senior figure said he could see nothing in my
records to indicate that my care or treatment was
inappropriate. However I wouldn't expect medical
people to write self-criticism in their notes. Dr. Callan
had died and could not be questioned about my illness.
I said I wasn't happy. I said my disablement and
unemployment three years after my treatment started
bore clear testimony to the failure of my treatment. A
consultant from another Trust concurred with the first
and I subsequently arranged to meet him, with an
'independent' NHS observer. I said that I had told my
GP of the urge to place my clenched hands in front of
my face before I was first referred to Dr. Callan – the
implications being that I was very seriously ill and
should not have been returned to a stressful job. The
first prescription was well short of the mark as I could
have received up to 80mg Bolvidon even as an
outpatient. And it was seven months before my
prescription was increased, during which I had gone
through inhuman and indescribable suffering. After
three years of treatment I was left unemployed and

disabled. He countered that he had not seen my GP's notes. (a cop out which I should have persued). He said that he agreed that my unemployment and disablement were a consequence of my original illness. But he did not really rationalize why this did not indicate medical negligence. He simply said that medicine is not an exact science and that anti depressants can take months to get into the system and achieve their full effect. I find this to be a wishy washy justification for the seven month delay in giving stronger medication. The fact that my medication was doubled is a clear indication of an inaccurate initial diagnosis. Why should I have had to wait seven months, enduring a horrific experience which drives people to suicide before reconsideration was made? Anything could have happened. He said that because I was prescribed anti depressants, because my prescription was (eventually) increased he could not conclude medical negligence. Of course Dr. Callans 'get rid of it easily enough' and 'only a bit of anxiety' comments were of no use because he was not around to confirm, explain or deny them. I said I was still not satisfied so my complaint was referred to the Complaints Convenor. A third (unknown) Psychiatrist I was later informed had concurred with the first two so the complaint could only progress to the Health Service Ombudsman. The Ombudsman could not however investigate clinical issues before 1995 and so I had nowhere else to go. I suppose it's naïve to expect a huge organisation to concede defeat to an undefended lone individual. Who pays these consultants? Why the NHS of course, the very organisation whom I would like to compensate me. I do still genuinely retain my beliefs that my treatment was botched and I note that psychiatric patients often commit suicide. There I rest my case. The first consultant who looked at my notes said that my treatment was 'entirely appropriate'. Perhaps when a patient under a psychiatrist stands in front of an express train he would find that 'entirely appropriate' too. It's pretty obvious to me that my treatment was botched. Doctors can be expected to make mistakes but when this happens patients ought to be entitled to redress. Not so it seems in the world of Psychiatry where it must be far easier to bury mistakes, negligence and sloppy work in the patients 'personality problems' or unfortunate circumstances.

In my view both my GP and Dr. Callan should have detected that I was seriously and dangerously ill. Instead I was given a relatively low dose of anti depressant, and returned to a highly stressful working environment when I was grossly incapacitated and horrifically ill. My medication was only reviewed after seven indescribable months. I was lost and bewildered in a dream, or should I say a nightmare. Anything could have happened. I received no protection and little support from other areas of the psychiatric/medical services. And after three years of medication, struggling in a working world only suited to those in health I was left disabled and potentially ruined for life despite making every effort to save my future. To this day Dr. Callan is and always will be in my mind the man who made a bungling error of judgement and in doing so condemned me to protracted suffering, long-term ruin and a shattered future. And he got away with it, along with all of the other medical people who I didn't find to be very good at what they did.

Concluding philosophy.

Young people tend to be naïve and gullible. Here are some of my mistaken beliefs at age 22:

That everything inside my head was 'me' and under my control.

That I was automatically going to die old.

That every problem could be overcome by rage and determination.

That people with mental problems could 'sort themselves out'.

That depression is about how people are feeling about life.

That I was special, and exempt from the worst things in life.

That humans are greatly different from animals.

That all Doctors are competent and caring.

That 'society' cares about me.

That I would always get a second chance if I screwed up.

Basically, through a lack of experience, my indoctrination into the human race and my religious upbringing, my head was full of magical thinking.

Lessons in life.

In summary, a combination of naivity, stupidity and bad luck took me to clinical depression. I am only guilty of one of these things. I suffered anxiety, stress and a breakdown in my social and nervous health. I was not to know about the lethal monster within my own head would be released when the threshold limits of anxiety are breached. This type of depression follows on from anxiety. It is the nature of the depression that is not understood. And even worse for the patient it's something nobody around them will understand. If I had read this book at age 19 or 20 I would never have gone through such a terrible and destructive experience. That has been a major inspiration for me to write it for the benefit of others. And I have written it because I felt tormented by the lack of understanding people showed about my illness and angry that the medical profession had failed to give me a second chance. Mental illness is common and people should be as aware of it as much as other common dangers. As a patient I hated the fact that nobody seemed to really know or understand my illness and this has been another inspiration. I hated reading through descriptions of depression in books and finding that they did not match up to what I came to feel sure about what had gone wrong.

To those who would avoidably put themselves in harms way in the belief that someone or something will protect them my advice is simple – don't. The world inherently weeds out individuals and isn't at all choosy. Anyone will do because every person who ever lived and ever will is merely another member of the species homo sapien. Nothing more. We are, beneath any hype, one race of stone age hunter gatherers on an exponential population growth curve. To those people who treat animals without respect because they have been indoctrinated to believe they are something totally different, please think again. We are all biological machines built by genes, biologically related and given just one shot at it. Being cruel and unnecessarily killing other living things is still a hideous immoral crime, even though they are not our species so we may never be brought to account for it.

Anyone of a religious persuasion will no doubt dislike some of the ideas in this book. I am not against private faith but I do not like to see people becoming slaves to religion, forming irrational and extreme views, allowing themselves to be manipulated by it or committing atrocities in it's name.

I hope this book has changed the reader's perception of the world for the better. And I hope it will stop other young people from making the awful journey I did. It was a very long way home and a journey some patients sadly will never make. If anyone is disturbed about having a terminator inside their head, just realise it is part and parcel of being a living thing in a mortal and dangerous world. It is intended as your best friend in

the worst circumstances. Just be aware that like a
hedgehog it hasn't caught up with the modern world.

www.ingramcontent.com/pod-product-compliance
Lightning Source LLC
Chambersburg PA
CBHW031215270326
41931CB00006B/565